The Complete Guide to Lifelong Nutrition

American College of Endocrinology

Co-edited by Jeffrey I. Mechanick, MD, FACP, FACE, FACN

and Elise M. Brett, MD, FACE, CNSP

Contributing Editor Donald A. Bergman, MD, MACE

ISBN: 1439270252
ISBN-13: 9781439270257

Acknowledgments

The editors thank Laurie Sund, MD, Certified Bariatric Physician, for her review of chapter 1.4. Healthy Eating.

The editors would like to thank Bryan Campbell, Director of Public and Media Relations, American Association of Endocrinologists, and Kate Mann, PharmD, Medical Editor, for their help in this project.

Contributors

Donald Bergman, MD, MACE
Clinical Professor of Medicine
Department of Medicine
Division of Endocrinology, Diabetes, and Bone Disease
Mount Sinai School of Medicine
New York, NY
Past President AACE
Past President ACE
Chair Power of Prevention Committee

Elise M. Brett, MD, FACE, CNSP
Associate Clinical Professor
Mount Sinai School of Medicine
Division of Endocrinology, Diabetes and Bone Disease
New York, NY

Himani Chandra, MD
Clinical Instructor, Mount Sinai School of Medicine
Division of Endocrinology, Diabetes, and Bone Disease
New York, NY

Arthur B. Chausmer, MD, PhD
Professor of Medicine (Adjunct)
Endocrinology and Metabolism
Johns Hopkins University School of Medicine
Baltimore, MD

Maria L. Collazo-Clavell, MD
Associate Professor of Medicine
Division of Endocrinology, Diabetes, Metabolism and Nutrition
Department of Internal Medicine
Mayo Clinic
Rochester, MN

Ayesha Ebrahim MD, FACP, FACE, FACN, CNS
Director of Endocrinology Services
Minnesota Center for Obesity, Metabolism and Endocrinology (MNCOME)
St Paul, MN

Martin M. Grajower, MD, FACP, FACE
Assistant Clinical Professor of Medicine
Albert Einstein College of Medicine
Private Practice
Riverdale Medicine, LLP
Riverdale, NY

J. Michael Gonzalez-Campoy, MD, PhD, FACE
Medical Director and CEO
Minnesota Center for Obesity, Metabolism and Endocrinology, PA (MNCOME)
Eagan, MN

Osama Hamdy, MD, PhD, FACE
Medical Director, Obesity Clinical Program
Joslin Diabetes Center
Assistant Professor of Medicine,
Harvard Medical School
Boston, MA

Jason M. Hollander, MD, CNSP
Endocrinology Associates of Princeton, LLC
Princeton, NJ

Daniel L. Hurley, MD Co-Chair, AACE Nutrition Committee
Department of Medicine and Division of Endocrinology, Diabetes, Metabolism, and Nutrition
Mayo Clinic
Co-Chair, AACE Nutrition Committee
Rochester, MN

Carol J. Levy, MD, CDE
Medical Scientific Director-Endo East
Novo Nordisk
Courtesy Faculty Weill Cornell Medical College
New York, NY

M. Molly McMahon, MD, MSc
Associate Professor of Medicine
Division of Endocrinology, Diabetes, Metabolism and Nutrition
Co-Chair, AACE Nutrition Committee
Mayo Clinic
Rochester, MN

Jeffrey I. Mechanick, MD, FACP, FACE, FACN
Clinical Professor of Medicine
Director, Metabolic Support
Division of Endocrinology, Diabetes and Bone Disease
Mount Sinai School of Medicine
New York, NY

Harriette R. Mogul, MD, MPH
Associate Professor
Director of Research, Division of Endocrinology,
Department of Medicine, New York Medical College
New York, NY

Philip Rabito, MD, FACE
Co-Director- Division of Endocrinology
Elmhurst Hospital Center
Assistant Professor of Medicine
Mount Sinai School of Medicine
New York, NY

Ronald Tamler, MD, PhD, MBA, CNSC
Director, Mount Sinai Men's Health Program
Assistant Professor, Division of Endocrinology, Diabetes, and Bone Disease
Mount Sinai School of Medicine
New York, NY

Michael Via, MD
Assistant Professor of Medicine
Albert Einstein College of Medicine
Beth Israel Medical Center
New York, NY

David A Westbrock, MD, FACP, FACE
Assistant Clinical Professor of Medicine, Wright State University
Boonshoft School of Medicine
Chief Executive Officer: New Profile Weight Management Center
Centreville, OH

Yi-Hao Yu, MD, PhD
Endocrinologist
Easton Endocrinology Associates
Core Teaching Faculty, Easton Hospital
Adjunct Faculty Member
Preventive Medicine and Nutrition
Easton, PA
Columbia University College of Physicians and Surgeons
New York, NY

Table of Contents

Part 4 - Nutrition for Specific Problems

Part 5 - Advanced Topics in Nutrition

Part 6 - Appendices

Foreword

Most people want to be successful and are willing to work to achieve that success. Most people also want to be healthy, but few are willing to work to sustain good health. This is because none of us is born successful, but most of us are born healthy. We assume we will continue to be healthy without any effort. Unfortunately, except for those who have inherited "longevity genes," most of us will have to strive to maintain the good health that was given to us at birth. From birth, factors programmed into our metabolism cause us to age and eventually to wear out. The good news is that healthy living (proper nutrition and physical activity) can forestall and, in some cases, prevent many chronic illnesses. This can allow us to age gracefully and lead productive lives well into our later years.

Eating carelessly can lead to weight gain, predisposing us to diabetes, high blood pressure, heart disease, some types of cancer, and premature aging. Poor eating habits can also lead to inflammation caused by "oxidative stress." When we eat, oxygen is needed to release energy from food. During this process, the oxygen is altered and becomes very reactive, combining with almost anything it contacts. This "free radical" oxygen is trapped by the body and disposed of; but if we eat unhealthy foods, some of this reactive oxygen escapes. This process causes inflammation and tissue damage, which can lead to heart disease, aging, and in some cases, cancer.

Proper nutrition and physical activity can help reverse this process. By eating the right foods and by engaging in daily physical activity, we can control excessive weight gain and oxidative stress, allowing us to live longer, healthier, and more productive lives.

The chapters in this book will explain the principles behind healthy eating and will provide you with specific recommendations about what to eat. Sections will deal with the prevention of illness, but will also address what you can do through diet if you already have diabetes, obesity, cardiovascular disease, osteoporosis, and other chronic illnesses.

This manual of nutrition is an important part of the American Association of Clinical Endocrinologists (AACE) and American College of Endocrinology (ACE) Power of Prevention campaign, which began in 2003. This program is for both adults and children and shows how each of us can achieve a healthy, long life through proper nutrition and physical activity.

I would like to thank the editors, Jeff Mechanick and Elise Brett. I would also like to thank Don Jones and the AACE/ACE staff including Bryan Campbell, as well as the chapter authors for a job well done.

The idea behind the Power of Prevention campaign is simple and straightforward: each of us, if we are given the right information, has the power to lead a long, healthy, productive life.

It has been said that to be successful, we need three things. We need information to develop our skills; we need reassurance that we are in good shape; and we need recognition and encouragement. This manual will help you get started with the first item in this list. The rest is up to you!

Donald Bergman, MD

Introduction

Jeffrey I. Mechanick, MD, FACP, FACE, FACN
Elise M. Brett, MD, FACE, CNSP

Nutrition is a common buzzword used in many casual as well as professional conversations regarding health care, lifestyle management, and simply the pleasures of routine living. But what exactly is nutrition? Webster defines it as: "the act or process of nourishing or being nourished; *specifically*: the sum of the processes by which an animal or plant takes in and utilizes food substances" (http://www.m-w.com/dictionary/nutrition).

From a practical standpoint, nutrition involves food, diets and meal plans, and ways in which people ingest, digest, and process foods. Food is necessary for life and should be enjoyed. Good nutrition can help promote a long, healthy life. Throughout history, eating has been a fundamental part of personal survival, togetherness, and cultural activity. Even the word *companion* is derived from the Latin *com* (meaning "with") plus *panis* (meaning "bread" or "food").

Foods, meals, and diets have changed based on availability of animals and plants, skills with agriculture, harvesting and hunting, the emergence of science and industry, cultural preferences, and other socioeconomic-political factors. As you will read, the transition from a diet based on whole foods, especially plants, to one that is based on processed grains and animal fats has been associated with increased risks for obesity, diabetes, and heart disease. "Healthy eating" is based on returning to a plant-based, whole food diet that is high in fiber, low in saturated animal fats, and "balanced" among nutrients.

Two very important problems with nutrition are undernutrition and overnutrition. Undernutrition, in our society, usually results from diseases that cause problems with swallowing, digestion, or absorption of nutrients as opposed to lack of access to food. Overnutrition, as in overweight or obesity, is a more common problem in America, and is observed not only in people who can afford lots of food but also in those with limited financial means who have easy access to inexpensive calorically dense food that is high in saturated fat, sugar, and salt. This is not just an "American" problem, but a global one as well, cutting across diverse ethno-cultural barriers.

It is not enough to "know" what to eat; one must have the resources available to implement a healthy diet. Indeed, the medical community needs to partner with the media, industry, government, schools, and the workplace to promote strategies that make healthy foods more affordable and available to everyone.

This book is organized into five broad parts. The first part, "Basic Knowledge in Nutrition," discusses general concepts like how to read a "Nutrition Facts label" and what exactly a healthy diet is. The second part is "What We Eat," which discusses the basic components of a healthy diet and wraps up with the culinary arts and what constitutes a healthy meal. The third part,

"Nutrition through the Life Cycle," discusses nutrition for children, pregnant and nonpregnant women, men, and the elderly. The fourth part is "Nutrition for Specific Problems"; it discusses nutrition and certain disorders such as diabetes, heart disease, obesity, and cancer. Here you will also find chapters on artificial nutrition, dietary supplements, and nutrition for the athlete. The fifth part is "Advanced Topics in Nutrition," which is geared for those readers with a specific interest in the physiology, biochemistry, and molecular biology of nutrition. Coursework in biology and chemistry at the high school level is necessary to capture the main points presented in these advanced topics. Finally, there are various reference tables at the end of the book, which can be referred to while reading the main text.

The Power of Prevention: The Complete Guide to Lifelong Nutrition follows *The Power of Prevention Guide to Physical Activity*, which was published by the American Association of Clinical Endocrinologists (AACE) and American College of Endocrinology (ACE) in 2006. The purpose of *this* nutrition guide is to provide a broad scope of topics geared to promote healthy eating that leads to a healthy lifestyle and can help prevent disease. One thread that will weave through the book begins with understanding what a healthy food is, then how to incorporate healthy foods into healthy meals, and then how to maintain healthy eating practices. This guide is presented in a language that is easy to understand so that the principles can be used in everyday life. General principles that affect almost everyone, as well as specific topics that affect only a few, are included. The chapters are short and not intended to cover an entire topic exhaustively, rather they just convey key practical "take-home" points.

What makes this book different, however, is that every single chapter is written by an "MD" who is an endocrinologist with expertise in nutrition and a member of AACE. The information contained in their chapters reflects not only an unbiased, objective, and scientific viewpoint, but also years of clinical experience from taking care of real patients with nutritional issues.

We recommend that you first look at the table of contents and identify chapters that interest you the most. For instance, if you are overweight and are concerned about having a heart attack, then chapter 4.7. "Nutrition and Heart Disease" would be a good starting point. However, if you have no real preferences and are simply interested in learning about healthy eating and improving your overall health, then just start at the beginning with "What Is Nutrition?" and continue the chapters in order, skipping any topics that are less appealing.

We hope that you learn some valuable tools from reading this book and have a little fun along the way. You may even wish to share this book with children, parents, other family members, and friends who may benefit from the information presented here. Eating is a necessary activity and should be enjoyed while also improving your chances for a long, healthy life. This book is designed to *empower* the reader to understand healthy eating and the specific ways to actually do it, not just for a few weeks or months, but for a lifetime.

Chapter 1.1

Nutritional Science, Public Health Nutrition Issues, and Key Definitions

M. Molly McMahon, MD

Nutritional Science

The history of nutritional science is ancient. In 400 BC, the Greek physician Hippocrates said, "Let food be your medicine and medicine be your food." Nutrition is a science that examines the relationship between diet and health. Nutrition is important to maintain health, prevent common medical conditions, and treat certain medical conditions. Nutrition affects each one of us in crucial ways. The Surgeon General's 1988 Report on nutrition stated that "for the two out of three adult Americans who do not smoke and do not drink excessively, one personal choice seems to influence long-term health prospects more than any other – what we eat."

Examples of Nutrition Public Health Issues

In January 2000, the Department of Health and Human Services launched Healthy People 2010, a comprehensive nationwide health promotion and disease prevention program. This program included goals to improve the health of all people in the United States during the first decade of the twenty-first century. The focus areas included nutrition, diabetes, and food safety, among others.

Public health nutrition issues that are discussed within this section apply to the general "healthy" population as well as those with specific nutritional issues. These issues include:

- the epidemic of obesity and type 2 diabetes in adults,
- obesity in children and adolescents,
- benefits of a plant-based diet as recommended by many national medical groups,
- food safety,
- an example of a common vitamin (D) deficiency that has unhealthy effects, and
- government bans of an unhealthy fat called "*trans* fat."

The Epidemic of Obesity and Type 2 Diabetes in Adults

Obesity is an epidemic in this country and a major public health issue. A drastic increase in weight gain and obesity has occurred in this country and around the world since the 1980s.

Approximately two-thirds of adult Americans are at least overweight, and about one-half of those people are obese. Obesity affects certain ethnic groups more than others, including African Americans, Mexican Americans, Native Americans, as well as people from lower socioeconomic classes.

As the incidence of obesity has increased, the likelihood of developing obesity-related diseases, including type 2 diabetes, heart disease, unhealthy levels of blood fats, high blood pressure, gastroesophageal reflux (heartburn), sleep disturbances, degenerative arthritis, and certain cancers, has increased. The disease risk of obesity becomes greater with increasing body mass index (BMI; see chapter 4.2, "Nutrition and Overweight-Obesity"). Quality of life of obese persons may also be adversely affected. Obesity is second only to tobacco as a cause of preventable death. Furthermore, obesity is costly. The cost is greater than the cost of smoking or problem-drinking.

This epidemic is caused largely by our culture, which promotes excessive food intake and discourages physical activity. We need to build a culture that makes it easier to buy reasonably priced healthy foods and to enjoy physical activity. Reaching this goal will require health-care providers, the food industry, schools, government, worksites, and the general public to work together.

The increase in obesity has resulted in an epidemic of type 2 diabetes (see chapter 4.1, "Nutrition and Diabetes"). Diabetes now affects nearly 10 percent of the US adult population and even higher numbers of Hispanic, Native American, and African American groups.

The Epidemic of Obesity in Children and Adolescents

In the last thirty years, the prevalence of being overweight among children between the ages of two and five years has doubled, and that of children and adolescents between the ages of six and nineteen years has tripled. About one in three children and adolescents is overweight (with a BMI in the 85th to 98th percentile for age and sex) or obese (with a BMI above the 95th percentile). Childhood obesity is associated with negative health consequences, including diabetes and risk factors for heart disease, such as high blood pressure and unhealthy levels of blood fats. In addition, the social discrimination experienced at this time in a young person's life can be devastating to his or her emotional well-being.

Factors contributing to increased caloric intake and decreased physical activity include large portion sizes, lack of family meals, soft drinks containing high fructose corn syrup, fast foods, power of food marketing to this age group, availability of labor-saving electronic devices, increased time spent watching television or playing video games, and decreased levels of physical activity, including decreased number of physical activity programs in schools.

Value of Plant-based Diets

Many national medical organizations recommend eating a plant-based diet. What is a plant-based diet, and what are potential health benefits? A plant-based diet is a diet rich in fruits, vegetables, whole grains, legumes (beans, peas, and lentils), and nuts, with smaller amounts of red meat and refined grains, such as white bread. Studies report that diets rich in fruits and vegetables can lessen the risk of obesity, diabetes, heart disease, stroke, cataracts, and macular degeneration (a disease of the eye); can decrease elevated levels of blood pressure and cholesterol; and can result in healthy bowel habits.

Fruits and many vegetables are low in calories and high in vitamins, fiber, and other beneficial nutrients. Current national dietary guidelines recommend at least nine servings of fruits and vegetables a day and preferably more. What are examples of one serving size? One serving of fruit is ½ cup sliced fruit, 1 small apple, 1 medium orange, ¾ cup blueberries, 2 small fresh figs, or ½ cup of most fruit juices. One serving of a vegetable is 1 cup broccoli, 1 medium tomato, 1 cup cauliflower florets, 1 cup cooked eggplant, or 2 cups of raw, leafy greens. It is best to choose a variety of different fruits and vegetables and a variety of colors.

It is also recommended to add in whole-grain breads, pastas, rice, oats, and cereals. Whole grains contain fiber and are an important source of vitamins and minerals. When reading product ingredient lists for whole-grain products, look for "whole grain" or "whole wheat" as one of the first ingredients in the list.

Food Safety and Prevention of Foodborne Illnesses

Avoiding foods contaminated with harmful bacteria, viruses, parasites, toxins, and chemical and physical contaminants is essential. Food poisoning, also called food borne illness, can result from eating contaminated food. One may develop gastrointestinal problems, like upset stomach, nausea, vomiting, and abdominal pain; fever; or dehydration. These issues can start just hours after eating the contaminated food. Food poisoning is particularly serious and potentially life-threatening for young children, pregnant women and their fetuses, older adults, and people with weakened immune systems.

E. coli bacterial infections have been in the news in recent years. E. coli are bacteria that live in the intestinal tract of healthy people and animals. Most of the bacteria are harmless and play a key role in absorbing certain vitamins. However, a few strains of E. coli are responsible for serious food-borne infections. A particularly dangerous strain of E. coli can cause severe bloody diarrhea, kidney failure, and even death. Most cases have been traced to eating undercooked ground meat, but the bacteria can also contaminate raw fruits and vegetables, such as lettuce, sprouts, tomatoes, spinach, and green onions.

Changes in food production during the past fifty years help explain the potential for organisms to cause food-borne illnesses. Many foods are produced in very large amounts and shipped to many states and markets. Infectious organisms can contaminate food at any point during its processing, cooking, or storage. Cross-contamination—the transfer of harmful bacteria from one surface to another—is often the culprit.

To help prevent food poisoning:

- Wash hands, utensils, and cooking surfaces often with warm, soapy water.
- Keep raw foods separate from ready-to-eat foods.
- Refrigerate or freeze perishable foods within two hours of purchase or preparation.
- Defrost food safely—not at room temperature but in the refrigerator, in the microwave, or under cold water.
- Cook foods to a safe temperature.

- Refrigerate foods quickly since cold temperatures keep harmful bacteria from growing and multiplying.
- Eat locally, when possible, to support local food growers and avoid food transportation delay and safety issues.

Vitamin D Deficiency as an Example of a Common Vitamin Deficiency

Vitamin D is one of the oldest vitamins known. Vitamin D is found in foods, like fortified milk and eggs, and in supplements. The sun also contributes to our daily production of vitamin D. Ten to twenty minutes of sun exposure each day can help prevent deficiency. Sunscreen use and skin pigmentation reduce vitamin D synthesis. Research reports that many people are vitamin D deficient. This is significant because new information shows how important vitamin D is for many body functions.

Vitamin D is important for absorption of calcium and phosphorus and to maintain strong bones. Recent information suggests that vitamin D may provide protection from osteoporosis, high blood pressure, cancer, and autoimmune illnesses. Vitamin D is very important for immune function as well.

Recommendations from the Institute of Medicine for adequate daily intake of vitamin D are 200 international units (IU) for children and adults up to fifty years of age, 400 IU for adults fifty-one to seventy years of age, and 600 IU for adults seventy-one years of age and older. However, most medical experts agree that most adults need far higher daily amounts. For most teenagers and adults, up to 2000 IU daily of vitamin D is safe and potentially beneficial. Doctors can measure the level of vitamin D in the blood and recommend the desired vitamin D dose.

Trans Fat and Government Bans

Trans fats, or partially hydrogenated vegetable oils, were developed early in the twentieth century as a cheaper alternative to animal fats. Food manufacturers like using *trans* fat because they help foods stay fresh longer and because they have a less greasy feel. Major sources of *trans* fat have included deep-fried fast foods, bakery products, prepackaged snack foods, margarines, and crackers.

Certain cities, like New York City, and countries, like Denmark, have banned *trans* fat use. Research has found that *trans* fat has unhealthy effects on blood fat levels and on the risk of heart disease. *Trans* fat increases levels of low-density lipoprotein cholesterol (LDL, or "bad cholesterol") and decreases levels of high-density lipoprotein levels (HDL, or "good cholesterol"). *Trans* fat also may contribute to heart disease by causing inflammation.

Since *trans* fat has no health value but does have risk, guidelines recommend eating less than two grams of *trans* fat a day. The government requires nutrition labels for all packaged foods to list the content of *trans* fat. However, foods containing less than 0.5 grams of *trans* fat per serving may claim to have 0 grams on the Nutrition Facts label. Therefore, reading the food label is important for foods carrying a *trans* fat-free icon to see if the product contains "hydrogenated" or "partially hydrogenated" fats. If it does, the product has small amounts of *trans* fat and it is better to choose another product without partially hydrogenated fats.

Some food manufacturers are substituting saturated fats for *trans* fat, but this will not solve the health problem. While *trans* fat is considered more harmful than saturated fat, too much of either increases the risk of heart disease and stroke. Food chemists are testing healthier cooking oils and fats to find replacements for *trans* fat that do not alter food taste or texture adversely.

Helpful Words and Concepts to Understand

There are many words and concepts that are used in discussions of foods, nutrition, and metabolism. These are listed in the glossary below and can be referred to as needed in the course of reading various parts of this book.

Antioxidants. Cellular metabolism requires oxygen, and this oxidation can produce reactive substances known as "free radicals" that can damage cells. For example, oxidative damage can cause cells to multiply and grow into a tumor, alter cholesterol-carrying particles in our blood, and damage protein in the lens and retina of the eye. Antioxidants are substances that slow down oxidative damage. Our bodies make some antioxidants, and we get some from the foods that we eat. Antioxidants are abundant in fruits, vegetables, nuts, and whole grains. Many antioxidants are identified by their colors: the red of cherries and tomatoes, blue of blueberries and grapes, orange of carrots and sweet potatoes, and green of collard greens, spinach, and kale. For instance, "carotenoids" include beta-carotene found in carrots and sweet potatoes; "lycopene" is found in tomatoes, watermelon, and pink grapefruit; "anthocyanins" is found in berries and plums; and "lutein" is found in green leafy vegetables, such as spinach and collard greens.

Basal Metabolic Rate (BMR). Also called basal energy expenditure (BEE), this is the amount of energy expended by an individual at rest. BMR can be measured by indirect calorimetry (a machine that analyzes respiratory gases) or can be estimated using equations based on age, height, weight, and sex, such as the Harris-Benedict Equation (see below). BMR decreases with loss of lean body mass and with increasing age. Building muscle through exercise increases BMR. Currently no medications are available that safely and effectively increase metabolic rate.

The Harris-Benedict equations to calculate BMR:
For men = 66.5 + (13.75 x kg) + (5.003 x cm) - (6.775 x age)
For women = 655.1 + (9.563 x kg) + (1.850 x cm) - (4.676 x age)

Daily Energy Expenditure, The calories needed in a day is determined by the basal metabolic rate (BMR), calories used during food digestion, and calories used during physical activity. In general, the BMR accounts for about two-thirds of our daily energy expenditure. Digesting, absorbing, and storing foods accounts for another 10 percent of daily energy (another word for calories) needs and does not vary greatly from person to person. The reminder is accounted for by calories burned in physical activity and for activities of daily living. This amount varies from person to person. It is best to be as active as possible so more calories are burned.

Obesity. An excess of body fat is the most common nutritional disorder in this country. Obesity is associated with medical conditions, including type 2 diabetes, high blood pressure, heart disease, abnormal amounts and types of blood fats, sleep disturbances, degenerative arthritis, and certain cancers.

Body Mass Index (BMI). BMI is an estimate of body fat and is associated with certain health risks. It is a formula that is determined by your body weight and height. BMI equals weight in kilograms divided by height squared (in meters). Medical experts suggest that underweight BMI is less than 18.5; normal BMI is 18.5 to 24.9; overweight BMI is 25.0 to 29.9; and obese BMI is 30 and greater. It is important for patients to know their BMI value.

Calorie (also kilogram calorie, kilocalorie, or kcal). A calorie refers to the amount of heat needed to raise the temperature of 1 kilogram of water by 1 degree Centigrade. Calories reflect the amount of energy—or fuel—provided by food. Carbohydrates, fats, and proteins are the nutrients that contain calories.

Dietary Reference Intake (DRI). We all need the same nutrients, but the amounts we need depend on age, sex, and a few other factors. For example, pregnant or breast-feeding women may need more of certain nutrients. DRIs are numbers that indicate how much of a certain nutrient are needed. They were established to prevent nutritional deficiencies and reduce the risk of common diseases such as osteoporosis, cancer, and heart disease. Terms associated with DRI can be confusing. There are four types of DRI reference values: estimated average requirement, Recommended Dietary Allowance, adequate intake, and tolerable upper intake level. The Recommended Dietary Allowance (RDA) is the more commonly recognized term. RDA refers to the average daily dietary intake level that is sufficient to meet the nutrient requirements of healthy people in a particular life stage and sex.

Energy Density. Energy density refers to the calories in a given amount of food. Foods high in fat have a high energy density. Foods high in water content and fiber typically have a lower energy density. In other words, low energy density foods have fewer calories in a larger amount of food. Fruits and vegetables are examples of low energy density foods, and ice cream and other confectionary desserts are examples of high energy density foods.

Macronutrients and Micronutrients. Nutrients are sorted into categories on the basis of their chemical structures and functions. Macronutrients are nutrients that are generally required in relatively large amounts. Macronutrients primarily include carbohydrates, proteins, and fat. In addition to other functions, macronutrients contain calories and are the body's main calorie source. Micronutrients refer to nutrients that are required in relatively smaller amounts. Micronutrients primarily include vitamins, minerals, and phytochemicals, which are discussed below. Micronutrients are very important but do not contain calories.

Malnutrition. Malnutrition generally results from a state of inadequate nutrition intake, increased requirements during certain illnesses, or changes in the body in very sick patients. With malnutrition, body stores of amino acids, the building blocks for protein, become less, and this can have adverse effects on health. Malnutrition may also refer to unbalanced overnutrition as seen with obesity.

Phytochemicals. Phytochemicals refer to a wide variety of compounds produced by plants. *Phyto* is the Greek word for plant. Phytochemicals are found in fruits, vegetables, and whole grains. Some act as antioxidants. Familiarity with some names is fun because you can recognize the value of certain foods. Examples include flavonoids, which are found in dark chocolate, fruits, vegetables, and tea; carotenoids, such as beta-carotene, lycopene, and lutein, which are found in red and yellow vegetables; phytosterols, which are found in nuts, seeds, whole grains, and plant oils; and isoflavones, which are found in soy products, beans, and legumes (beans, peas, and lentils).

Eating more fruits, vegetables, whole grains, and legumes can reduce your risk of certain cancers and heart disease and is better than relying on dietary supplements. The bottom line is to eat fruits and vegetables of different colors to gain health benefits as they may help prevent conditions such as heart disease, diabetes, cancer, and cataracts. Phytochemicals are very important nutrients and are believed to contribute to the colors, textures, smells, and tastes of fruits and vegetables.

Selected References

American Association of Clinical Endocrinologists Power of Prevention. "Nutrition." http://www.powerofprevention.com/nutrition.php (accessed on October 18, 2008).

American Heart Association. "Diet and nutrition." http://www.americanheart.org/presenter.jhtml?identifier=1200010 (accessed on October 18, 2008).

Center for Nutrition Policy and Promotion, US Department of Agriculture. "Dietary Guidelines for Americans 2005." http://www.healthierus.gov/dietaryguidelines (accessed on October 18, 2008).

Harvard School of Public Health. The nutrition source: vegetables and fruits. http://www.hsph.harvard.edu/nutritionsource/fruits.html. Accessed January 23, 2008.

MayoClinic.com. "Food and nutrition." http://www.mayoclinic.com/health/food-and-nutrition/NU99999 (accessed on October 18, 2008).

Chapter 1.2

Nutrition Facts Label

M. Molly McMahon, MD

The United States government requires that food manufacturers provide nutrition information on food labels to help people purchase, prepare, and eat healthier foods and proper amounts of food. Food labels provide several different types of information, including serving size, nutrition facts, a listing of ingredients, and nutrition and health claims (see figure, page 14).

Starting at the Top of the Nutrition Facts Label

Labels tell you much of what you need to know about what is contained in food. The label shows the serving size. The serving size is a specific amount of food defined by standard measurements such as cup, ounce, or piece. The label also lists calories per container so you can determine the content per package.

At a minimum, the following nutrients are listed based on one serving of the food item:

- **Total calories and calories from fat** indicate how much "energy" is in the food
- **Total fat** – fats and oils are a source of energy for the body
- **Saturated fat** is found in foods of animal origin such as meats, poultry, dairy, and eggs; saturated fat increases total and LDL ("bad") cholesterol
- ***Trans* fat** is a fat type that can increase the risk of heart disease
- **Cholesterol** is found in foods of animal origin; the body also makes cholesterol to build cells; cholesterol is a substance in fatty deposits (plaques) that can develop in blood vessels; plaque buildup can reduce blood flow in your blood vessels
- **Sodium** is the major component of "salt"
- **Total carbohydrates** are not only sugars but also include starches and fiber
- **Dietary fiber** is found in whole foods, fruits, vegetables, whole grains, and legumes, such as peas, beans, and lentils; fiber is a very healthy nutrient
- **Sugars** can make a food sweet
- **Protein** is the building blocks of our cells
- **Vitamins A and C** are important for various metabolic functions in our bodies and can be found in many fruits and vegetables
- **Calcium** makes our bones strong but is also important for many other body functions
- **Iron** is necessary for our red blood cells to carry oxygen

In general, one should limit the intake of nutrients listed at the top of the Nutrition Facts label, including total fat, saturated fat, *trans* fat, cholesterol, and sodium, and eat more of the nutrients listed on the bottom of label, including fiber, vitamins A and C, calcium, and iron. Too much or too little of any nutrient can potentially have an adverse effect on overall health.

What Does Daily Value (DV) Mean?

For most nutrients listed, there is a daily value (DV), a dietary goal, and percent DV (DV divided by the dietary goal). These values are listed on the label to the right of the specific nutrient. The DV numbers tell you how much of the daily recommended amount of nutrients are contained in one serving of the food. These percentages are based on a usual dietary goal of 2,000 calories a day. By following the dietary suggestion, a person can stay within the recommended upper or lower limit for the nutrient listed, based on a 2,000-calorie diet. For many people, however, healthy eating may require more or less than 2,000 calories. For instance, most people who are trying to lose weight need to stick to a healthy eating plan that limits calories to less than 2,000 per day. On the other hand, some people, such as those who are underweight or have certain medical problems or burn excessive amounts of calories through exercise or are very tall, may need to eat more than 2,000 calories per day. The point here is that the nutritional information is "based" on a 2,000-calorie diet, and if you eat more or less, the information needs to be adjusted for you.

- Five percent DV or less is considered "low."
- Twenty percent DV or more is considered "high."
- If a person eats more or less than 2,000 calories per day, then the percent DV can still be used as a frame of reference. If the label space permits, the footnote will sometimes include percent DV based on a 2,500-calorie diet.
- No daily reference value is listed for sugar because no recommendations have been made for the total amount to eat in a day. People should compare similar products (such as different breakfast cereals) and then try to choose a product that is lower in sugar content. Other names for added sugars include high fructose corn syrup, corn syrup, sucrose, glucose, maple syrup, and fructose.
- Percent DV is required for protein only if a claim is made for protein, such as "high in protein" or if the food is meant for use by infants or children under four years old.
- *Trans* fat has no percent DV.

Nutrient Intake Guidelines

Below the asterisk at the bottom of the label is a list of key nutrients. The amount of recommended key nutrient intake is based on the total caloric intake. For example, if a person eats a 2,000-calorie diet, then the amount of fat consumed each day should be less than 65 grams. This means that if only 20 grams of fat are in one serving of a product, then 45 grams of fat may be consumed during the rest of the day.

So, how much of these nutrients should be consumed each day, based on a 2,000-calorie diet?

- Total fat: less than 65 grams
- Saturated fat: less than 20 grams
    - o There is no DV for *trans* fat.
    - o The FDA and American Heart Association recommend keeping *trans* fat intake as low as possible and preferably under 2 grams per day.
- Cholesterol: less than 300 milligrams
- Sodium: less than 2,400 milligrams
- Total carbohydrate: less than 300 grams
- Fiber: at least 25 grams

Foods Without Nutrition Facts Labels

Some foods do not have Nutrition Facts labels. These include:

- vegetables, fresh fruits, and bulk items—there may be a handout or display in the store providing such information for these items;
- fish, meat, and poultry—ask the grocery store staff for nutrition information since some producers will voluntarily label these foods and follow governmental guidelines.

Ingredient Listing

Ingredients are listed below the Nutrition Facts label in descending order by weight. The first ingredient is the predominant one in that food.

Nutrient and Health Claims

Food labels may carry other information. For instance, they may state that the product is a good source of a particular nutrient. Products also may claim to benefit a certain condition or to alter the risk for certain medical conditions, including heart disease, cancer, or osteoporosis. Manufacturers are not required by law to carry nutrient or health claims. However, if claims are made, they are regulated by the government and must be backed up by scientific evidence.

Label Definitions

The government also regulates the use of certain phrases and terms on product labeling. These include the following and their specified definitions.

- *Free*: this means that the product is absolutely free of the nutrient, or if the nutrient is in the food, the amount must be insignificant.
- *Light*: must have half the fat or one-third fewer calories than the regular product. *Light* can also mean that the sodium content of a food has been reduced by at least 50 percent

compared with the regular product.

- *Low*: the food can be eaten frequently without exceeding dietary guidelines for fat, saturated fat, cholesterol, sodium, or calories. However, terms can be misleading. "Low fat" does not necessarily mean "low calorie," so check out the total calories too and compare similar products to choose the healthier one.
- *Reduced*: food must contain at least 25 percent less of a nutrient in terms of calories than the regular product. However, note that the regular product may be very high in calories, sodium, and fat, so the "reduced" product may not necessarily be a healthy choice.

Moving Beyond Food Labels

The terms *fortified* and *enriched* mean that nutrients have been added to the food. Specifically, *fortified* means that nutrients were added that were not originally present, and *enriched* means that nutrients lost during processing were replaced. Fortifying and enriching foods helps eliminate nutritional deficiencies that used to be common.

Examples of fortified foods and the nutritional illnesses they help prevent include:

- Salt. Potassium iodide was added to salt to help prevent an enlarged thyroid (goiter) that may result from iodine deficiency.
- Milk. Vitamin D was added to milk to help prevent rickets, a bone disease that results from insufficient vitamin D.
- Breakfast cereals. Many are fortified to provide approximately 25 percent of most daily micronutrient requirements.
- Grain-based foods. Folic acid is added to grain-based foods (bread, cereal, pasta, and rice) to help meet nutrient needs and reduce the chance of birth defects and possibly heart disease.
- Fruit juices. Some are fortified with calcium to increase daily calcium intake and improve bone health.

Examples of enriched foods include:

- Flour. Refining flour removes certain nutrients, so flour is often enriched with iron and B vitamins. Flour and foods made with flour (breads, pasta, and cereals) became enriched at the start of World War II to help nourish troops.
- Pasta enriched with folic acid.

Take-home Points

People should use Nutrition Facts labels and ingredient listings to help select healthier foods. At first, labels and ingredient listings can seem confusing, but a little information and practice reading labels can equip a person with the tools and confidence to make healthy nutrition choices. Remember that it is not only what you eat at one time, but also what you eat over the course of the day, week, and month that ultimately results in healthy nutrition habits. Foods should be compared in order to select the healthiest choice within a particular food group. If certain foods do not have Nutrition Facts labels, then look for store handouts or displays for nutrient information. Finally, healthy foods should also taste great.

Selected References

American Heart Association. "Reading food labels." www.americanheart.org/presenter.jhtml?identifier=3046050 (accessed on October 18, 2008).

MayoClinic.com. "Nutrition facts: Reading the food label." www.mayoclinic.com/health/nutrition-facts/NU00293 (accessed on October 18, 2008).

Planning Meals. In: Rizza R, Go W , McMahon M, Harrison G, eds. "Encyclopedia of Foods: A Guide to Healthy Nutrition" San Diego, CA. Academic Press; 2002.

US Food and Drug Administration. "How to understand and use the Nutrition Facts label." www.cfsan.fda.gov/~dms/foodlab.html (accessed on October 18, 2008).

Nutrition Facts

Serving Size 1 cup (228g)
Servings Per Container 2

Amount Per Serving

Calories 250 Calories from Fat 110

	% Daily Value*
Total Fat 12g	**18%**
Saturated Fat 3g	**15%**
Trans Fat 3g	
Cholesterol 30mg	**10%**
Sodium 470mg	**20%**
Total Carbohydrate 31g	**10%**
Dietary Fiber 0g	**0%**
Sugars 5g	
Protein 5g	
Vitamin A	**4%**
Vitamin C	**2%**
Calcium	**20%**
Iron	**4%**

* Percent Daily Values are based on a 2,000 calorie diet. Your Daily Values may be higher or lower depending on your calorie needs.

	Calories:	2,000	2,500
Total Fat	Less than	65g	80g
Sat Fat	Less than	20g	25g
Cholesterol	Less than	300mg	300mg
Sodium	Less than	2,400mg	2,400mg
Total Carbohydrate		300g	375g
Dietary Fiber		25g	30g

See text, page 9

Chapter 1.3

Living a Healthy Life

David A. Westbrock, MD, FACP, FACE

Three important aspects of a healthy lifestyle are healthy eating, physical activity, and adequate sleep. All three must work together in order to truly create a healthy lifestyle.

Healthy Eating as Part of Healthy Living

Eating a balanced, healthy diet is essential to healthy living. Integrating the right amounts of fruits, vegetables, and whole grains into your diet each day will provide proper nutrition to keep your body running and your energy up. Good nutrition also does something else: it makes you feel good. Consuming a lot of processed foods tends to lower energy levels and deprives your body of the essential vitamins it gets from healthy, wholesome foods.

Healthy eating pertains not only to what you eat but how much. Controlling portions is extremely important when trying to eat healthy. Overeating even the healthiest foods can contribute to excess weight or make weight loss difficult. Many times, portions, or serving sizes, are overestimated, resulting in additional calories. For example, one serving of dry pasta is ½ cup, which is about what fits into an ice cream scoop. That is substantially smaller than the size of a pasta dish at most restaurants. Think about how many servings are in a typical overflowing bowl of spaghetti. Of course, all people are different and, therefore, have different daily caloric needs. People should check with their doctors about how many calories they actually need in order to achieve and then maintain a healthy weight.

Get Moving

One of the numerous misconceptions about exercise is that it has to be difficult and last a long time in order to make it count. That is not necessarily true. Simply put, we just need to start moving. However, to truly make a lifestyle change, we need to start by changing our attitudes toward exercise. Changing the way we think about exercise is one of the most important steps to making sure it becomes a habit.

Think about how much physical activity you get in any given day. Is it ten minutes? Thirty minutes? Is it any at all on most days? Physical activity must become a habit in order to lose or maintain weight. The Centers for Disease Control (CDC) recommends that individuals get thirty minutes of moderate activity on most days of the week or twenty minutes of vigorous activity three times a week. The Dietary Guidelines for Americans, available on the Web at http://www.health.gov/dietaryguidelines/dga2005/document/html/chapter4.htm, advises thirty minutes of moderate-intensity physical activity above a normal routine on most, if not all, days of the week. This can reduce the likelihood of developing a chronic disease. If greater health benefits or weight loss are desired, then even more physical activity, perhaps sixty minutes extra a day, is advised.

Why is increased physical activity healthy? Think about our bodies and what they were designed for. Tens of thousands of years ago, we needed to be active constantly. Whether hunting or being hunted, we needed to keep moving to stay alive. Watching TV or sitting behind a desk at work does not support our engineering.

One way to increase physical activity is to do things differently. There are simple ways we can trick ourselves into being more active. Here are some examples:

1. Take the stairs instead of the elevator.
2. Choose a parking spot that is far away from your destination.
3. If you have ten- to fifteen-minute blocks of time several times during the day, take several ten- to fifteen-minute walks.

Most people who are just beginning to exercise start with a simple walking routine. Walking is a low-impact, effective way to increase your fitness level and transition to higher levels of activity and is an exercise that is more important than our "too busy to exercise" excuses. It can be done relatively anywhere with minimal equipment. Walking is always convenient. You can leave your desk and walk around your building or up and down the stairs; you can walk out the front door of your house; you can walk in a mall; and you can walk from your faraway parking spot, bus stop, or train station.

Pedometers are small inexpensive devices that can be worn on a belt or shoes that measure the distance you walk or run. They are useful tools that not only keep track of your activity but also serve as a subconscious motivator. If you wear one, chances are you will be checking your activity throughout the day and trying harder to reach your goal of increasing your activity.

Obesity

If you are obese, part of achieving a healthy lifestyle involves weight loss through behavioral change. There is currently no cure for obesity. As much as we all want to hear that a magic pill has been invented that will allow us to eat whatever we want, as much as we want, without exercising, well, we might as well be wishing on a star. True, there are amazing scientific advancements that allow us to treat terrible diseases and disorders, but obesity is one that will keep coming back unless we do one thing: change our lifestyles. Many people know that losing weight does not mean the battle is over—that is the easy part. If you are truly committed to being at a healthy weight, losing weight is just the beginning. It is *maintaining* weight loss that is the ongoing battle. Simply defined, we must truly change the way we incorporate food and activity into our lives—forever.

Why a lifestyle change instead of just a diet? No fad diets can claim that they have the proprietary key to long-term weight loss. It is vital for people who want to lose weight and become healthy to adopt a healthy lifestyle for one reason: it is the only thing that works. Yes, people do lose weight all the time on fad diets, but again, that is the easy part. The tough part is keeping it off. If you lose weight and then go back to the same habits that you had before, obviously the weight will come back.

Ain't Misbehavin'

Chronic diseases such as hypertension, diabetes, and high cholesterol are not generally curable, but can remain under control with lifestyle changes in addition to medication. If you have one of these conditions or are at risk for one of these conditions, you will need to change the way you eat and exercise in order to stay healthy. In other words, you can help yourself to stay healthy. When looking at whether you have truly changed your behaviors to reflect a healthy lifestyle, ask yourself the following: Am I eating a healthy, balanced diet most of the time? Am I exercising on most days?

Keep Yourself in Check

The first step in changing your eating habits is to keep track of everything you eat. Yes, everything. So often people mindlessly throw food into their mouths and do not even realize how much they consume. It is often helpful to keep a "food journal" or "food diary" documenting everything you eat. After a while, new habits are developed in which food is consumed with more thought and appropriate restraint where needed. If you are trying to lose weight, this also helps to tally daily caloric intake.

It takes a long time to change old habits, but this can be facilitated by having a strong support network. That might mean keeping up with an organized weight management program or finding friends who share similar ideas about good health. If you typically eat with a spouse or companion, it can be helpful to receive dietary counseling together and/or make changes together.

Beware of the Weight Loss Wreckers

There are many things that can sabotage efforts to be healthy (see Sabotage Alerts), including attitudes, actions, and sometimes even other people. Once people are aware of what can ruin their efforts, they will be better equipped to deal with them and continue on a healthy path.

Overall, achieving a healthy lifestyle requires commitment, dedication, and a true understanding that being healthy is only temporary unless behaviors are changed. Chronic illnesses and many other medical disorders may not be curable, but to the extent that there is a nutritional component to their cause or behavior, such conditions may be preventable and managable with healthy lifestyle changes.

Sabotage Alerts

Sabotage Alert #1: *The notion that this should be easy.* Some people think that if they begin down a healthy path and are not perfect every step of the way, they have failed. Learning a new lifestyle is not easy. If it were, more people would do so and we would not have an obesity epidemic on our hands. Understand that there will be good days and bad days. The difference lies in what is done after the bad days. After a bad day, one should move on, not throw away all the good work that has been accomplished, and not go back to old habits.

Sabotage Alert #2: *Negative attitudes.* The truth is that a person's own determination is the only thing he or she can truly count on. Negative thoughts and the "I can't do this" attitude are normal, but they can also ruin efforts to become healthier. Taking responsibility for one's own actions and developing a positive outlook are very important to long-term success.

Sabotage Alert #3: *Sleep deprivation.* Sleep involves the production of two hormones: "ghrelin," which stimulates appetite, and "leptin," which sends signals to the brain when enough food has been eaten. It is very interesting that both of these hormones play a role in the way a body's fat composition and food intake communicate with the brain. When a person does not get enough sleep, the body produces more ghrelin, which stimulates the appetite, and less leptin, which causes him or her to feel less satisfied after eating. When tired, most people tend to crave sugary, high-calorie, nutrient-deficient foods—and lots of it. When sleepy, a body's defenses are down and less likely to make healthy choices. It is important to get the proper amount of sleep when learning a healthy lifestyle. Additionally, when well-rested, there is more energy to be active and exercise.

Suggested Readings

American Association of Clinical Endocrinologists. *Power of Prevention Guide to Physical Activity.* AACE, 2006.

Centers for Disease Control and Prevention. "Healthy Living." http://www.cdc.gov/HealthyLiving/ (accessed on November 2, 2008).

Center for Nutrition Policy and Promotion, US Department of Agriculture. "Dietary Guidelines for Americans 2005." www.healthierus.gov/dietaryguidelines (accessed on October 18, 2008).

MayoClinic.com. "Healthy Living." http://www.mayoclinic.com/health/HealthyLivingIndex/HealthyLivingIndex (accessed on November 2, 2008).

National Heart Lung and Blood Institute. "Tipsheet" http://nhlbisupport.com/chd1/Tipsheets/sevenways.htm (accessed on August 2, 2008).

Chapter 1.4

Healthy Eating

J. Michael Gonzalez-Campoy, MD, PhD, FACE

The days of being on a "diet" are over! The focus now is on *healthy eating*. Instead of focusing on foods that you cannot have and worrying about food intake, look for foods that you should eat. Instead of dreading the next meal and how you may give in to temptation, make eating and sharing the mealtime experience with others a simple pleasure, like it was intended. Healthy eating is important, both for maintaining good health and for preventing disease. For health, it is important to emphasize that pretty much everything in moderation is good. To prevent disease, meals should provide the necessary raw materials, fuels, and additives the body needs. Healthy eating is what good nutrition is all about!

The human body is just like a car. Every cell in the body must be refueled to function properly. The human body must also have access to spare parts and additives. All of these come from what we eat. The stomach and intestines break down foods into building blocks. These building blocks are then absorbed from the gut into the circulation and delivered to the tissues by the blood.

There are three major sources of fuel and building blocks for the body; these are known as macronutrients:

- Proteins
- Carbohydrates
- Fats

Digestion breaks down protein into amino acids, carbohydrates into simple sugars like glucose, and fat into triglycerides. In addition to macronutrients, our bodies also get micronutrients from what we eat. Micronutrients are needed in small quantities for life and include vitamins, minerals, certain electrolytes, and other plant-derived compounds, including herbs, which are called "phytonutrients." Think of micronutrients as the additives, like oil and wiper fluid, that your car needs to function properly.

What we eat may also contain substances that are harmful to the body. Poisons are the most obvious case. Bacteria and viruses that can cause infections are another example. The excessive consumption of foods that may otherwise be healthy and essential is a third example. This last category includes the excessive consumption of salt (sodium), which may worsen hypertension and accelerate bone loss, and of calories, which leads to obesity.

The term *malnutrition* is the opposite of healthy eating. Malnutrition occurs when one does not have access to enough food ("undernutrition") or when one consumes too much food ("overnutrition"). Poor food choices may lead to the consumption of excess calories and the development of overweight or obesity. In the setting of overweight or obesity, deficiencies in vitamins, minerals, and protein can develop.

Nutritional deficiencies cause disease. This is why Recommended Dietary Allowances (RDA) were introduced by the Food and Drug Administration (FDA) in the United States. The Dietary Reference Intakes (DRI, see appendix 6.1.) are the values most recently established by the FDA for use in official nutrition labeling. Healthy eating should include the use of dietary supplements when the DRI values are not met with meals alone.

Regularly Scheduled Meals

Your car runs better when you service and refuel it regularly. Your body works better when you feed it at regular intervals. Modern humans are genetically engineered to survive famine. Long times without food, or skipped meals, change your metabolism and drive you to consume more calories when you do eat. If you are overweight or obese, you should strive to have well-balanced meals spaced throughout the day to avoid excessive consumption of calories or insufficient intake of nutrients.

Every time you eat, your body has to spend calories to digest the meal. Therefore, regularly scheduled meals lead to regular activity of the gut. When the gut is working regularly, the body enters a healthy state for fuel economy. Only a small meal, such as a piece of fruit, is required to get the digestive process going.

The Caloric index of Food

The caloric index of foods is the amount of energy that is contained in each of the major macronutrients:

- Protein provides 4 calories per gram.
- Carbohydrate provides 4 calories per gram.
- Fat provides 9 calories per gram.

It follows that 1 gram of fat gives you more than twice the number of calories than 1 gram of carbohydrate or protein. High-fat foods are "calorie dense" and, therefore, excessive consumption of fats increases the chance of becoming overweight or obese. As a general rule, fats that are liquid at room temperature, especially plant oils, are better than fats that are solid at room temperature. Also, solid fats usually contain *trans* fats, which increase the risk for heart disease. Lard, butter, margarine, and peanut butter are best when consumed in restricted amounts. Animal products are also rich in saturated fats, which leads to an increase in blood cholesterol levels, a major risk factor for heart disease.

There are sources of calories other than macronutrients. For example, alcohol yields 7 calories per gram, but does not support the nutritional needs of the body. These are called "empty calories," and they go to producing fat tissue rather than energy that can be used by the whole body. Sweetened carbonated beverages are another source of empty calories. Choosing only non-caloric beverages when you are thirsty will help prevent the consumption of excess calories.

Conversely, when you eat foods that have high water content, you ingest fewer calories. It is recommended to eat at least seven to ten servings of fruits and vegetables every day. Fruits and vegetables are a good source of fiber. Fiber can help distend the stomach wall and create a sensation of fullness. If you eat a large salad for an appetizer, you may consume fewer calories for the meal than if you start with a roll and butter. Of course, one needs to be careful to limit calories from the salad dressing, which is typically high in fat. However, you do not need to feel hungry (no "dieting") when eating in a healthy way.

The "Plate Method"

The "plate method" also helps you eat healthy. First, divide your main plate into quarters. Two quarters should be for vegetables, preferably lightly steamed without added fat. One quarter of the main plate should be for meat and protein. A good rule of thumb to follow is that the meat portion should be about the size of a deck of cards. Lean cuts of meat, fish, and poultry without the skin are preferred. Red meat should be limited due to its high saturated fat content. The last quarter of your main plate is for starch or carbohydrate. Carbohydrate choices that are not processed; that also contain fiber, vitamins, or protein; and that do not require added fat for preparation are generally the best. For example, a baked potato with the skin is a better choice than mashed or fried potatoes. Whole grains such as quinoa, bulgar wheat, or brown rice are better choices than white rice. Whole-grain pastas, breads, and rolls are better than white. Beans are always an excellent carbohydrate choice as they are high in fiber and also contain protein.

In the Idaho Plate Method depicted in the figure (see page 23), two additional smaller plates are used. One is for fresh fruits and the other for low- or no-fat dairy products, such as fat-free or low-fat milk, cottage cheese, or yogurt. Another modification to help with portion control would be to use salad plates. Varying foods for different days, different meals (breakfast, lunch, or dinner), and dessert items (fresh fruit or yogurt) can make eating healthy meals more interesting.

Food Preparation and Storage

Many of the foods we eat in industrialized countries are processed. This means that they are chemically changed from their natural condition. They can be canned, wrapped, packaged, bottled, frozen, refrigerated, dehydrated, refined (as with white bread or pasta), or otherwise treated in an aseptic (free of bacteria) way. Foods that are processed generally contain preservatives, and frequently this causes them to lose their nutritional value. When you consume fresh fruits and vegetables, you receive the full nutritional value of these foods.

Viruses, bacteria, and fungi are everywhere, including in the food we eat. To a large extent, when foods go to waste it is because these infective agents have used the food for themselves and have grown on it. Many foods must be refrigerated or frozen to prevent these infective agents from growing. Cooking food is good to kill bacteria and for palatability, but bad because fiber is degraded and phytonutrients are lost (the green water after boiling spinach, for instance).

Healthy eating involves getting the highest nutritional value from food, while minimizing the risk of infection from contamination. The risk for infection from what we eat is predictably higher in some specific circumstances. For example, eating raw shellfish carries a risk of infection with the hepatitis A virus. Those foods that carry an infectious risk should be well cooked to minimize that risk. Most meats and eggs should be thoroughly cooked. Fruits and vegetables should be washed with water. Good hand washing is very important prior to the preparation of any meal.

There are some recognized toxicities in some foods. For example, mercury levels have been reported to be very high in some fish and shellfish. Regular consumption of these foods may lead to toxic levels in children, pregnant women, or mothers who are nursing. The following links will provide you with more information on this subject: http://www.epa.gov/waterscience/fish/advice/ and http://www.cfsan.fda.gov/.

Roles of Snacks (Healthy Snacks)

Snacking can lead to excessive caloric intake, particularly when the snacks are calorie-dense. We can choose not to snack, but modern society provides easy access to food. Too much of the feeding we do is unnecessary. It is best to avoid being in situations where you are tempted to ingest food when you are not hungry.

Encourage those around you to eat healthy also. Fruits and vegetables are examples of healthy, low-calorie snacks. Consider bringing a plate of fruit to your next staff meeting or recreational activity instead of doughnuts, pastries, or other high-fat and sugar-containing foods. Instead of mid-morning snacks, organize mid-morning walks to boost energy. Be a positive role model for good nutrition and a healthy lifestyle!

Social Context of Meals

There truly is no such thing as good food or bad food. Once digested, all foods are turned into protein, carbohydrate, and fat. At the end of the day, what matters is the energy balance—how ingested calories compare to spent calories—and that you get the nutrients you need for health. A positive energy balance, when caloric intake is higher than caloric expenditure, leads to storage of calories as fat, and weight gain. A negative energy balance, when caloric intake is lower than caloric expenditure, leads to using more calories from fat, and weight loss.

Meals are an opportunity for healthy eating and creating bonds with those around you. Sitting down to a good meal is one of the greatest pleasures in life. And if you have good company, this helps to improve your lifestyle. Signals from the gut to the brain like the degree of stomach distention or the amount of peristalsis (the forward propelling movement of food by the intestines) can be delivered over time to cause a feeling of fullness. A meal that you eat by yourself may be consumed faster than the fullness signal takes to decrease hunger. This puts you at risk for ingesting more calories than you should. If you take your time, such as during a meal shared with others with interesting conversation, you may consume less and avoid overeating. If you must eat "on the run," then try to make an effort to eat more slowly. Making time to consume meals leisurely is an integral part of healthy eating.

Suggested Readings and Web sites to Browse

Center for Nutrition Policy and Promotion, US Department of Agriculture. "Dietary Guidelines for Americans 2005." www.healthierus.gov/dietaryguidelines (accessed on October 18, 2008).

Hensrud, DD. *Mayo Clinic Healthy Weight for Everybody*. Mayo Clinic, Rochester MN, 2005. Nutrition.gov. http://www.nutrition.gov (accessed on September 21, 2008).

Rinzler, CA. *Nutrition for Dummies*. Wiley Publishing, Inc., Hoboken NJ, 2006.

Sizer, F, Whitney E. *Nutrition: Concepts and Controversies, Tenth Edition*. Thomson-Wadsworth, Belmont CA, 2006.

United States Department of Agriculture, Center for Nutrition Policy and Promotion. http://www.cnpp.usda.gov (accessed on September 21, 2008).

United States Department of Agriculture, National Agriculture Library. http://fnic.nal.usda.gov (accessed on September 21, 2008).

Willett WC, Skerrett PJ. *Eat, Drink, and Be Healthy: The Harvard Medical School Guide to Healthy Eating*. Free Press, New York, 2001.

World Health Organization. "Nutrition." http://www.who.int/nutrition/en/ (accessed on September 21, 2008).

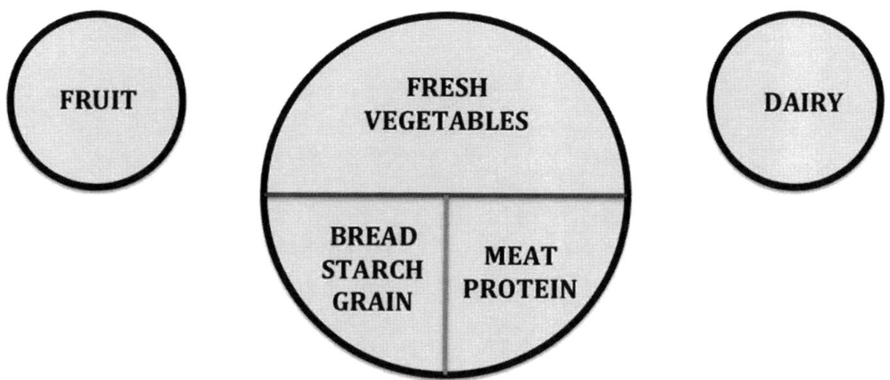

(http://www.cdc.gov/pcd/issues/2007/jan/06_0050.htm, accessed on September 21, 2008).
See text, page 21

Chapter 1.5

Ethnic and Cultural Aspects of Nutrition

J. Michael Gonzalez-Campoy, MD, PhD, FACE
Ayesha Ebrahim, MD, FACE

Food Is a Reflection of Our Heritage.

We are truly a global society. With the advent of modern communications, information and images from around the world are available in real time. Geographical barriers have been overcome by modern methods of transportation; people can travel around the world in a matter of hours. We all are able to experience many different cultures, and with this comes a great variety of foods.

There have been waves of immigrants entering the United States dating back to the first Pilgrim colonies. Each immigrant group has enriched our nation and added its culture, values, and cuisine. According to the US census, approximately 33.5 million foreign-born people lived in the United States in the year 2003, representing 11.7 percent of the US population. People born in Latin America comprised approximately 53.3 percent of the US foreign-born population in the year 2003. Every time we incorporate an immigrant group into our society, we benefit from their contributions. The Hmong and Vietnamese immigrants who came to our country in the 1960s and 1970s, and the Russian immigrants who have joined us since the end of the cold war, all add to our choices of meals. Indeed, the United States is a melting pot of cultures, backgrounds, and cuisines.

Meals bring people together and are frequently a central focus of religious or celebratory gatherings. Perhaps the best example in the United States is the Thanksgiving holiday, for which most of us prepare a turkey as the main part of the meal. Sharing a meal brings us together at births, weddings, graduations, and funerals. These special gatherings frequently allow us to reflect on our cultural background and perpetuate traditions unique to each of us. Whether you are Hindu and avoid beef; Muslim and fast for Ramadan or avoid pork; Jewish and eat kosher foods; or Christian and give up some foods for Lent, meals are an expression of your religious heritage as well.

Thus, food represents culture, geography, history, and religion. We have the opportunity to turn each meal, regardless of its origin, into a healthy eating experience! Table 1 demonstrates a few examples of healthy eating using ethnic foods.

The Joy of Food—The Senses and Relationships

A good meal is a pleasure to eat. Foods that are visually appealing, smell good, and taste great provide us with joy. The senses truly expand on the simple process of ingesting nutrients.

Simply, we need to ingest protein, carbohydrate, fat, vitamins, and minerals in adequate quantities to maintain good health. The social context of meals, on the other hand, is more complex. We all learn who to eat with, what to eat, how much to eat, and where to eat. Taste is acquired and learned. For most of us, meals shared with family and friends build pleasant memories. A date involves sharing a meal most of the time and business deals are frequently negotiated over food. When we host a meal, we feel the need to provide our guests with food until they are satisfied. Doing so is a reflection on us—our financial success when we can afford a nice meal, and our willingness to provide for those we care about. The time spent in the preparation of a meal and in consuming it is an investment in relationships. However, we must be diligent to make each meal a healthy experience!

In industrialized countries, the learned behaviors surrounding meals have drastically changed over the decades. We have gone from meals prepared at home, where eating brought the family together, to meals often consumed on the run and outside the home. We have also gone from freshly made meals to ready-to-eat meals that incorporate processed or preserved food.

Largely, these patterns of how we eat reflect how our society is evolving. When the automobile came along, suburbs developed, and as a result, we spend longer times commuting to work. At the same time, distances are less of an obstacle to pursue activities we are interested in. We have less time at home and less time to prepare our own meals. Therefore, we have relied on "fast food" and meals that require little preparation. The restaurants that are common in every city provide us with choices of food at various prices. This variety of sights, smells, and tastes is good, yet these choices also represent an erosion of our cultural background and limit the time spent with friends and family.

Additionally, the thought that we must "get our money's worth" has led to increasingly bigger portions of food we purchase. In some areas of the country, a successful restaurant must have such a large meat portion that it actually hangs over the edge of a large plate to show how much food one gets. Over time, both the larger portions and the high caloric density of restaurant foods have contributed to the epidemic of obesity in the United States. The choice of place to eat, therefore, must represent a balance between pleasing the senses, protecting the pocketbook, and eating healthy.

The nutritional value of foods decreases when they are not fresh. Most foods that are canned, wrapped, packaged, or bottled contain preservatives. With electricity and the implementation of freezers, food can be stored for longer periods of time. The use of both preservatives and freezing robs our foods of their freshness. And, in general terms, freshness gives foods better nutritional value. Those of us who eat at home and spend time preparing meals must face the fact that there is a price to pay for freshness. This, of course, involves frequent trips to the grocery store.

Healthy eating must involve a balance between eating out and eating in, processed food and fresh food, and food consumed on the run and meals shared with family and friends.

Genetics

Our genes are very important in determining our response to meals. The health benefits and risks we experience with our modern meals are genetically programmed. As an example, the "thrifty gene hypothesis" states that modern humans have genes that make them very effective at getting and storing calories. Many years ago, during times of famine, people who survived had genes that allowed them to pack away calories during times of plenty. On the other hand, those who did not have those genes died during the famines. Over the course of centuries, evolution has selected humans with these genes.

When a person moves from a society where portion sizes are restricted to a society that is exposed to larger portion sizes, these thrifty genes may not be so beneficial. In the presence of excess calories, the person starts putting away calories in the form of excess fat. Some people develop disease as a consequence of this accumulation of stored calories. Diabetes, hypertension, and high cholesterol values are examples of metabolic problems that are genetically programmed and show up with weight gain. People from the Asia and the Indian subcontinent are at higher risk for the development of these metabolic problems because they can develop them even without excess fat. Genetics are important in determining our response to our environment, which includes our meals.

Modern science is able to use genetics for the good of mankind. The scientist Thomas Malthus predicted that the planet earth had a limited capacity to produce food and that population growth would be restricted by the availability of food. Malthus never dreamed that we could bioengineer crops that would give higher yields per acre, or animals that could be bigger, or milk that could last longer. So populations have continued to grow around the world, and in most places, we have been able to provide food for them. There is, however, significant inequality in the distribution of foods around the world, with regions of famine that still exist.

Conclusion

Ethnic foods have tastes and sensations we may not be accustomed to. They can be incorporated into healthy meals by using the principles of healthy eating discussed in this book. For instance, ethnic dishes can be selected that contain plenty of fresh fruits and vegetables, with interesting and new herbs, spices, and other ingredients that are high in fiber and low in saturated fat and sugar. In this way, another dimension to healthy eating is realized: that eating food can be fun and adventurous.

Suggested reading

About.com. "Home Cooking: Ethnic Recipes and Foods." http://homecooking.about.com/od/ethnicrecipesandfoods/Ethnic_Recipes_and_Foods.htm (accessed on September 21, 2008).

Carnegie Mellon University. "Ethnic dishes." http://www.cs.cmu.edu/~mjw/recipes/ethnic/ethnic.html (accessed on September 21, 2008).

GourmetSpot. "Ethnic foods." http://www.gourmetspot.com/ethnicfoods.htm (accessed on September 21, 2008).

United States Census Bureau. http://www.census.gov (accessed on September 21, 2008).

United States Department of Agriculture, National Agriculture Library. http://fnic.nal.usda.gov (accessed on September 21, 2008; type in "ethnic" in Search FNIC field).

Table. Healthy Choices in Ethnic Foods

Chinese

- Steamed
- Jum (poached)
- Kow (roasted)
- Shu (barbecued)
- Steamed rice

Italian

- Red sauces
- Primavera (no cream)
- Piccata (lemon)
- Crushed or sun-dried tomatoes
- Lightly sautéed
- Grilled

Mexican

- Spicy chicken or fish
- Black beans
- Salsa or picante
- Soft corn tortillas
- Dishes that are not fried or breaded

Adapted from: The National Heart, Lung, and Blood Institute in cooperation with the National Institute of Diabetes and Digestive and Kidney Diseases, National Institutes of Health.

Chapter 2.1

Carbohydrates

Daniel Hurley, MD

What Are Carbohydrates?

Carbohydrates are sugars, starches, and fiber. Sugars and starches are the body's main energy sources and are found in many foods. The basic building block of carbohydrates (*hydrates* of *carbon*) is the sugar molecule, a simple union of carbon, hydrogen, and oxygen. Starches and fiber are complex connected chains of sugar molecules.

Carbohydrates are the most abundant of the four major types of nutrient molecules, which also include proteins, lipids, and nucleic acids. The primary role of carbohydrates is the storage and transport of energy as glucose, starch, and glycogen. The digestive system handles all carbohydrates in much the same way by breaking them down (or, in the case of fiber, trying to break them down) into single sugar molecules small enough to enter the bloodstream. It also converts most digestible carbohydrates into glucose (blood sugar), the universal energy source for the body's cells. The simple sugar, glucose, is required to satisfy the brain's energy needs. Muscle also uses glucose for energy for short bouts of activity. Sugar and starch are stored in the skeletal muscle and liver as glycogen, a reserve form of energy that can be called upon later for bodily needs.

Types of Carbohydrate

Dietary carbohydrates can be grouped into two main categories:

- Simple
    - Monosaccharides (one sugar molecule)
    - Disaccharides (two sugar molecules)
- Complex
    - Oligosaccharides (a few sugar molecules)
    - Polysaccharides (many sugar molecules)

Some of the biochemistry of carbohydrates will be discussed here, but a more detailed description of the biochemistry of nutrition is provided in chapter 5.1. Simple sugars were once considered "bad" and complex carbohydrates "good," but the real picture is much more complex.

Simple Carbohydrates

The simplest and most basic carbohydrate unit is called a monosaccharide. Monosaccharides cannot be broken down into simpler sugars. Monosaccharides make foods taste sweet. Examples of monosaccharides include glucose, fructose (natural fruit sugar), galactose, xylose, and ribose. Monosaccharides are the major source of fuel for the body and are used both as an energy source (glucose) and in the production of new molecules in a cell. When monosaccharides are not needed by cells, they are quickly converted into another form, such as polysaccharides.

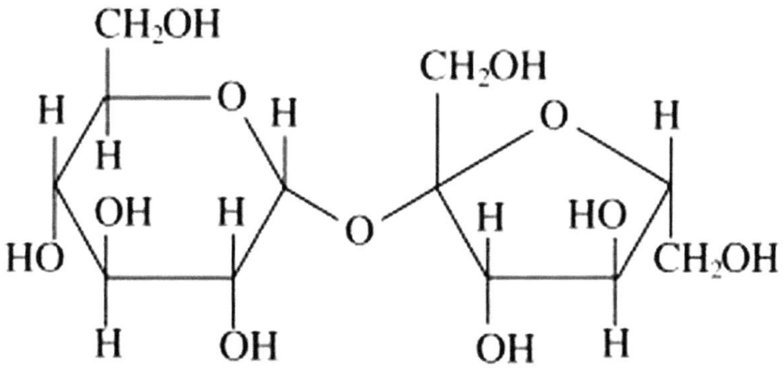

A disaccharide is a simple sugar (carbohydrate) composed of two monosaccharides. Examples of disaccharides include sucrose (common table sugar) and lactose (milk sugar).

Sucrose (above) is the most common disaccharide and consists of two monosaccharides, glucose (left) and fructose (right).

Complex Carbohydrates

These include molecules made of three or more linked sugars. Oligosaccharides and polysaccharides consist of long chains of monosaccharides that are bound together. Oligosaccharides typically contain three to nine monosaccharides, while polysaccharides contain ten or more monosaccharides. Polysaccharides function in either cell structure or energy storage. In plants, polysaccharides are stored as starch (amylose and amylopectin) and fiber, whereas in animals, polysaccharides are stored as glycogen (structurally similar but more densely branched). Glycogen is stored in the liver and muscle and can be metabolized easily to provide energy quickly for active body tissue metabolism.

Advantages and Disadvantages for Certain Carbohydrates

The most important carbohydrate is glucose, which is easily metabolized by nearly all living organisms. Plants create carbohydrates by photosynthesis, which can then be consumed by humans and used as fuel for cells. Many carbohydrate-containing foods (such as whole grains, vegetables, legumes, and fruits) are also rich sources of vitamins, minerals, and phytochemicals. After ingestion by humans, plant starch is digested and metabolized into simple sugars to generate 4 calories per gram, whereas plant fiber provides no calories.

Of the three macronutrients, carbohydrates are much simpler to metabolize than fats or proteins and, therefore, provide a more available short-term energy reserve. However, the strong affinity of carbohydrates for water makes bodily storage of large quantities of carbohydrates inefficient. Energy obtained from carbohydrate metabolism takes the form of "ATP" (adenosine triphosphate: the currency of energy in our bodies).

Dietary Sources for Each Type of Carbohydrate

Carbohydrates come from a wide variety of foods including breads, pasta, beans, bran, rice, cereals, potatoes, corn, soft drinks, milk, cookies, and many others.

Here are some suggestions for adding healthy carbohydrates to the diet:

- When shopping for cold cereal, check the label ingredient list and choose whole wheat, whole oats, or other whole-grain cereals; check the amount of fiber per serving and choose cereals with 3 to 5 and even up to 7 to 10 grams of fiber per serving.
- Eat whole-grain breads. Whole-grain products are labeled as whole grain, whole wheat, or rye. In contrast, bread products labeled as "made with wheat" (cracked wheat, seven-grain, multigrain, stone ground wheat) contain mostly refined flour and, therefore, do not have the nutrient benefit of whole-grain foods. Again, you can check the grams of fiber per serving to help select a "high-fiber" brand.
- Choose whole wheat pasta and brown rice instead of white pasta and rice. Try less familiar foods such as bulgur, wheat berries, millet, hulled barley, and quinoa.
- Eat beans. Beans are an excellent source of slowly digested carbohydrates and fiber, and also a great source of protein.
- Choose fresh fruit for dessert or snacks instead of baked goods.
- Have a vegetable salad as a starter for dinner or add a protein to a large salad for a complete lunch.
- Have a baked potato or yam instead of fried or mashed potatoes.

Impact on Obesity, Glycemic Control, and Diabetes

The Institute of Medicine recommends that adults consume between 40 and 65 percent of dietary calories from carbohydrates. The Food and Agriculture Organization and World Health Organization recommend a goal of 55 to 75 percent of total energy from carbohydrates, but only 10 percent of this total from "free sugars" (simple carbohydrates).

Obesity

The distinction between "good carbs" and "bad carbs" is an important attribute of low-carbohydrate diets. These diets have a higher fat content and promote a reduction in the consumption of grains and starches. They also contain less fiber and phytonutrients, which are components of healthy eating.

Some commercial low-carbohydrate diets use the term *net carbs*. This refers to the carbohydrates that are available for metabolism and specifically do not include fiber. This essentially allows the increased consumption of fiber in a low-carbohydrate (low-net-carbohydrate) diet.

The proposed theory of low-carbohydrate diets is important to understand. This theory is based on a reduction in insulin levels used to metabolize sugars and a suppression of hunger from fat metabolism. Some popular diets treat all carbohydrates as evil and the cause of all weight gain and body fat (e.g. the original Atkins diet). Indeed, the data tends to support that low-carbohydrate diets may result in quicker weight loss than low-fat diets, although research studies do not show benefits beyond one year.

In two short (six-month) "head-to-head" research studies on diets, low-carbohydrate (high-fat) diets resulted in more weight loss than low-fat (high-carbohydrate) diets. In a longer (twelve-month) study, overweight women (who have not undergone menopause) were given one of four diets: Atkins, Zone, Ornish, or LEARN (a standard low-fat, moderately high-carbohydrate diet). All women steadily lost weight during the first six months, with the most rapid weight loss occurring in the Atkins (low-carbohydrate) group. During the last six months of study, most women regained weight. At the end of one year, women in the Atkins group had lost more weight than the others (Atkins, approximately 10 pounds; LEARN, approximately 6 pounds; Ornish, 5 pounds; and Zone, 3.5 pounds). Blood levels of triglycerides, LDL-cholesterol ("bad" cholesterol), and HDL-cholesterol ("good" cholesterol) were at least as good in the Atkins group as those of the other diets.

It is of interest in this study that few women actually followed their assigned diets. The Atkins group ate almost three times more carbohydrates than assigned (50 grams per day); the Ornish group ate about 30 percent of total calories as fat (goal: less than 10 percent); and there were similar deviations in the Zone and LEARN diet groups.

What can be learned from these and other diet comparison studies? First, during a weight loss diet, calorie restriction is more important than the diet itself It is not the carbohydrate intake *per se* that causes weight loss (i.e., a "calorie is a calorie"), but rather a reduced intake of calories. Second, no one knows the long-term effects of limiting carbohydrates in the diet. Carbohydrate food sources contain a host of vitamins, minerals, and phytonutrients that are essential for good health, and their intake may be inadequate on a low-carbohydrate diet. Equally worrisome is the inclusion of excessive amounts of unhealthy fats in a low-carbohydrate diet and the potential risk of disease involving blood vessels. A large twenty-year research study of women looked at the relationship between low-carbohydrate diets and heart disease. Women who consumed low-carbohydrate diets that were high in vegetable sources of fat or protein had a 30 percent lower risk of heart disease. However, women who ate low-carbohydrate diets that were high in animal fats or proteins did not have a reduced risk of heart disease.

Glycemic Index and Diabetes

The glycemic index (GI) classifies carbohydrates based on how quickly and how high they boost blood glucose compared to eating simple sugar. Foods with a high GI, like white bread, cause a rapid spike in blood glucose. Foods with a low GI, like whole oats, are digested more slowly and result in a lower and slower change in blood glucose. Foods with a score of greater than 70 are defined as having a "high GI," and those with a score of less than 55 have a "low GI."

Diets rich in high GI foods cause quick and strong increases in blood glucose and have been linked to an increased risk for obesity, type 2 diabetes, and heart disease. Lower GI foods have been shown to help control type 2 diabetes and improve weight loss in some studies. Other studies have not found a GI effect on body weight or health. Thus, the true value of the GI remains to be determined.

Factors that influence the GI of carbohydrates include the following:

- *Type of starch.* Carbohydrates come in many different forms, and some starches are easier to break down into sugar molecules than others.
- *Processing.* One of the most important factors that determine a carbohydrate's GI is how much it has been processed. Milling and grinding removes the fiber-rich outer bran and the vitamin- and mineral-rich inner germ, leaving mostly the starchy endosperm. In addition, finely ground grain is more rapidly digested than more coarsely ground grain and, therefore, has a higher GI. When possible, replace highly processed grains, cereals, and sugars with minimally processed whole-grain products.
- *Fiber content.* The more fiber a food contains, the less digestible it is, thus limiting the sugar content delivered from the carbohydrate.
- *Ripeness.* Ripe fruits and vegetables tend to have more sugar and a higher GI than unripe ones.
- *Meal fat and acid content.* The more fat or acid a food or meal contains, the slower its carbohydrates are metabolized to sugar.

A limitation of the GI is that it does not define how much digestible carbohydrate a food delivers. For example, a Snickers candy bar has a low GI of 41, but it is far from being labeled a health food. The sweet-tasting watermelon has a very high GI but has only a small amount of carbohydrate per serving because watermelon consists mostly of water.

A new method to classify foods, called the "glycemic load," is based on the amount of carbohydrate in a given food and its impact on the blood glucose level. Thus, a food's glycemic load is determined by multiplying its GI by the amount of carbohydrate it contains. In general, a glycemic load of greater than 20 is high, 11 to 19 medium, and less than 10 low.

Dietary Fiber

Fiber refers to carbohydrates that cannot be completely digested and, therefore, pass through the intestine partially undigested. Fiber adds bulk to the diet, creates a sense of satiety (feeling "full" faster), and helps to control body weight. Fiber is present in all edible plants including fruits, vegetables, grains, and legumes. However, not all fiber is the same.

One way to categorize fiber is by its source of origin. For example, fiber from grains is referred to as cereal fiber. Another way to categorize fiber is by how easily it dissolves in water. Soluble fiber partially dissolves in water, whereas insoluble fiber does not dissolve in water. Insoluble fiber, as found in whole-wheat bread and brown rice, increases stool bulk, helps prevent constipation, and may reduce the risk of colon cancer. Soluble fiber, such as that contained in vegetables, fruit, and especially legumes, slows stomach emptying, reduces the rise in blood sugar after a meal, and reduces blood cholesterol levels.

Diets rich in soluble fiber and complex carbohydrates have been associated with improvements in blood fats, blood pressure, heart disease, and some types of cancer. The risk of developing type 2 diabetes reportedly declined by 30 percent in a study where men consumed greater than 8.1 grams of cereal grain fiber daily, compared to those eating less than 3.2 grams daily. Similar results have also been reported in women. Diets high in soluble fiber may improve glycemic control in patients with type 2 diabetes.

Current recommendations suggest that children (beyond one year) should consume at least 19 grams and adults 21 to 38 grams of dietary fiber daily, although the typical American adult averages only 15 grams of dietary fiber a day. The following may help to increase dietary fiber intake:

SOLUBLE FIBER	INSOLUBLE FIBER
Oatmeal	Whole grains
Oatbran	
	Whole grain breads
Some nuts and seeds	
	Barley
Legumes	
	Brown rice
Beans	
	Whole-grain cereals
Dried peas	
	Wheat bran
Lentils	
	Vegetables
Fruit	
	Carrots
Apples (pulp)	Celery
Blueberries	Cucumbers
Pears	Tomatoes
Strawberries	Zucchini

- Eat at least 4 to 5 cups per day of fruits and vegetables. Examples of fruits that are high in fiber are apples, oranges, berries, pears, figs, and prunes. Vegetables that are high in fiber include broccoli, cauliflower, brussels sprouts, green peas, carrots, and beans.
- Replace white bread with whole-grain breads.
- Choose brown rice instead of white rice.
- Consume other good sources of fiber such as bran, oatmeal, multiple-grain cereals (cooked or dry), and popcorn.
- Check labels on food packages for the listed amounts of dietary fiber.

Fiber may cause abdominal bloating, cramping, or gas. These symptoms may be prevented by introducing a small amount of fiber into the diet and slowly increasing that amount over time. Drinking water (nine 8-ounce glasses daily for women and twelve 8-ounce glasses daily for men) will help to digest fiber.

Suggested References

Center for Nutrition Policy and Promotion, US Department of Agriculture. "Dietary Guidelines for Americans 2005." www.healthierus.gov/dietaryguidelines (accessed on October 18, 2008).

Harvard School of Public Health. "The nutrition source." http://www.hsph.harvard.edu/nutritionsource/index.html (accessed on September 30, 2008).

MayoClinic.com. "Healthy living." http://mayoclinic.com/health/HealthyLivingIndex/HealthyLivingIndex/ (accessed on September 30, 2008).

National Center for Complementary and Alternative Medicine. http://nccam.nih.gov (accessed on September 30, 2008).

University of Sidney. "Home of the Glycemic Index" http://www.glycemicindex.com/ (accessed on September 30, 2008).

U.S. Department of Agriculture. MyPyramid.gov. http://mypyramid.gov (accessed on September 30, 2008).

Chapter 2.2

Fats

Daniel Hurley, MD

Fat Basics

Fat is an essential macronutrient that plays many roles in helping the body function properly. Fat is used as an energy source and in the production of cell membranes and hormone-like compounds called "eicosanoids." Eicosanoids help regulate blood pressure, heart rate, blood vessel constriction, and blood clotting. Dietary fat provides a sense of fullness after meals. Fats are also important as transport carriers for fat-soluble vitamins (A, D, E, and K) as they move from digested food in the intestine into the bloodstream and then to cells throughout the body.

Fat is a rich source of energy (9 calories per gram), and eating too much fat can be harmful. Eating high-fat foods can add excess calories and lead to weight gain and obesity. Even if body weight is maintained, eating too much of certain types of fats, such as saturated fats or *trans* fats, can increase blood cholesterol levels and the risk of coronary heart disease.

Fat Types

Most foods contain several different kinds of fats, such as saturated fats, polyunsaturated fats, monounsaturated fats, and *trans* fats. Fats are simple molecules that are classified by the chemical structure of their component parts. "Fatty acids" are molecules arranged in a line, or a chain, and are called "hydrocarbons." They are made of carbon (C), hydrogen (H), and oxygen (O). Fats, carbohydrates, and protein all contain carbon and are, therefore, "organic."

Four common classification systems exist for fatty acids. Three of them use the carbon atom chain length (usually 12–18) and the number and positions of any double bonds present. There are also two broad types of fatty acids: saturated and unsaturated. Saturated fatty acids have several hydrogen (H) atoms, which are from water, and all the linking bonds between the carbon (C) atoms are single (shown as single lines between the Cs).

```
  H H H H H H H H H H H H H H H H H    O
  | | | | | | | | | | | | | | | | |   //
H-C-C-C-C-C-C-C-C-C-C-C-C-C-C-C-C-C-C
  | | | | | | | | | | | | | | | | |   \
  H H H H H H H H H H H H H H H H H    OH
```

Stearic acid, a saturated fatty acid

Fatty acid chains with one or more double bonds that link carbon (C) atoms are "unsaturated" (either mono- or poly-unsaturated). Here, there are fewer hydrogen (H) atoms, and the fatty acid bends at the site of the double bond. This affects the shape, function, and metabolism of the fatty acid.

Monounsaturated fatty acids (MUFA) have one double bond.

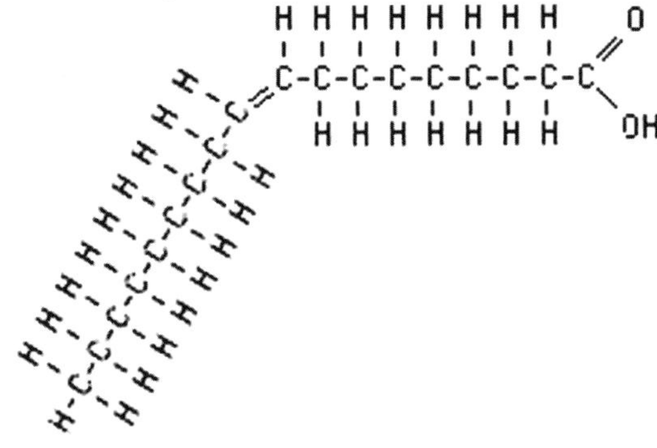

Oleic acid, a monounsaturated fatty acid. Note that the double bond is *cis*; this is the common natural configuration.

Polyunsaturated fatty acids (PUFA) have two or more double bonds.

Linoleic acid, a polyunsaturated fatty acid. Both double bonds are *cis*.

Triglycerides are formed when fatty acids are attached to a "glycerol" backbone. Triglycerides represent the major constituent of "dietary fat." When food is digested, fatty acids are released from the glycerol backbone and absorbed into the bloodstream.

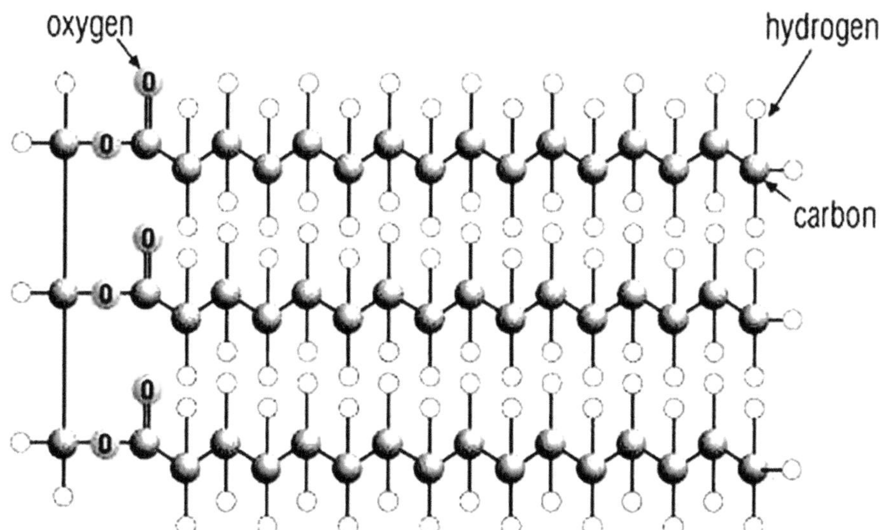

Cholesterol is an important part of a healthy body because it is used to produce cell membranes and certain hormones called steroids: estrogen (female hormone), testosterone (male hormone), cortisol (stress hormone), and many others. Cholesterol is a fat-like material present in foods from animal sources. Our bodies also make cholesterol. Dietary cholesterol and other fats are "oils" that have to be attached to a carrier protein in the liver before circulating in the blood.

When considered together, these fats and proteins are referred to as "lipoproteins." The major lipoproteins important for health are very low-density lipoproteins (VLDL), low-density lipoproteins (LDL-cholesterol, or "bad" cholesterol), and high-density lipoproteins (HDL-cholesterol, or "good" cholesterol) (see chapter 4.6, "Nutrition and Blood Fats").

LDL-cholesterol is the major cholesterol carrier in the blood. If too much LDL-cholesterol circulates in the blood, it can move slowly into the artery wall. This creates a fatty collection or "plaque," which then can narrow the inside of the artery. As a result, there is decreased blood flow to the brain (cerebral or carotid arteries), heart (coronary arteries), kidneys (renal arteries), and/or legs (peripheral arteries). This disease process is generally known as "atherosclerosis." A blood clot ("thrombus") that forms at a cholesterol plaque can narrow or block arterial blood flow and then cause an increase in blood pressure, a heart attack, or a stroke. LDL-cholesterol is known as "bad" cholesterol because a high LDL-cholesterol level is associated with atherosclerosis.

HDL-cholesterol accounts for about one-third to one-fourth of the blood cholesterol. HDL-cholesterol carries cholesterol from the body's arteries through the bloodstream to the liver, where it is metabolized and eliminated from the body. HDL-cholesterol is known as "good" cholesterol because a high HDL-cholesterol level is associated with a decreased risk of atherosclerosis.

Healthy Fats and the Mediterranean Diet

It is not necessary, or even desirable, to eliminate all fats from the diet. Instead, one should consume foods that contain healthier types of fats, such as unsaturated fats. Intake of unsaturated dietary fats, such as MUFA and PUFA, can lower the risk of heart disease by reducing the total and LDL-cholesterol blood levels.

Unsaturated fats are a big part of the healthy eating basics of the "Mediterranean diet." In particular, olive oil is the major fat source used in the traditional cooking and eating style of countries bordering the Mediterranean Sea. In studies in which MUFA and PUFA were eaten in place of carbohydrates, LDL-cholesterol levels decreased and HDL-cholesterol levels increased. These changes in blood fats are associated with a lower risk for a first heart attack. In addition, the Mediterranean diet has been shown to significantly reduce the risk of further heart disease in individuals who have already had a heart attack. Key components of the Mediterranean diet include:

- eating lots of fruits and vegetables daily (this can range from five to over ten servings a day depending on the particular Mediterranean diet: Greek, French, Italian, Spanish, or others);
- consuming healthy fats, such as olive oil and canola oil;
- consuming very little red meat;
- eating fatty fish twice a week (for example, salmon, lake trout, albacore tuna, mackerel, and herring);
- eating small portions (palm-sized amount) of nuts at meal or snack time; and
- drinking red wine in moderation.

In general, the Mediterranean diet is very similar to the American Heart Association's Step-I diet, but it contains less cholesterol and has more omega-3 fatty acids (defined below). Fish, a source of omega-3 fatty acids, is eaten on a regular basis. Sources of fat include olive oil, canola oil, and nuts, particularly walnuts. The Mediterranean diet limits saturated fats and hydrogenated oils (*trans* fats), both of which contribute to heart disease. Bread is a staple of the diet, but bread is eaten without butter or margarines, which contain saturated fats or *trans* fats.

Dietary Sources of Fat

Fats are a necessary part of a healthy diet. In other words, it is not healthy simply to "avoid all fat." However, what is important for healthy eating is to be aware of which fats are healthier than others. Therefore, in this section, fats are discussed in two broad categories: those that are relatively "good" for you, and those that may be "bad" for you.

Good Fats

MUFA and PUFA are good, or healthy, fats. These unsaturated fats are found in plant products such as vegetable oils, nuts, and seeds.

MUFA remain liquid at room temperature but may start to solidify in the refrigerator. Foods high in MUFA include olive, peanut, and canola oils. Avocados and most nuts also have high amounts of MUFA.

PUFA are usually liquid at room temperature and in the refrigerator. Foods high in PUFA include vegetable oils, such as safflower, corn, sunflower, soy, and cottonseed oils.

Omega-3 fatty acids are PUFA found mostly in seafood. Good food sources of omega-3 fats include fatty, cold-water fish, such as salmon, mackerel, and herring. Flaxseeds, flax oil, and walnuts also contain omega-3 fatty acids. Small amounts of omega-3 fats are also found in soybean and canola oils. (See figure)

The American Heart Association recommends that all adults eat fish, especially fatty fish. Potentially harmful contaminants (such as dioxins, mercury, and polychlorinated biphenyls or PCBs) are found in some species of fish and may be harmful to pregnant or nursing women. It is best for a pregnant/nursing woman to discuss these dietary concerns about eating fish with her doctor. In general, shark, king mackerel, swordfish, tilefish, orange roughy, marlin, and grouper have the highest concentrations of mercury and should be avoided with pregnancy or nursing. Smoked seafood and raw shellfish should also be avoided with pregnancy and nursing due to infection and contamination issues (see American Pregnancy Association Web site http://www.americanpregnancy.org/pregnancyhealth/fishmercury.htm and http://www.americanpregnancy.org/pregnancyhealth/foodstoavoid.html).

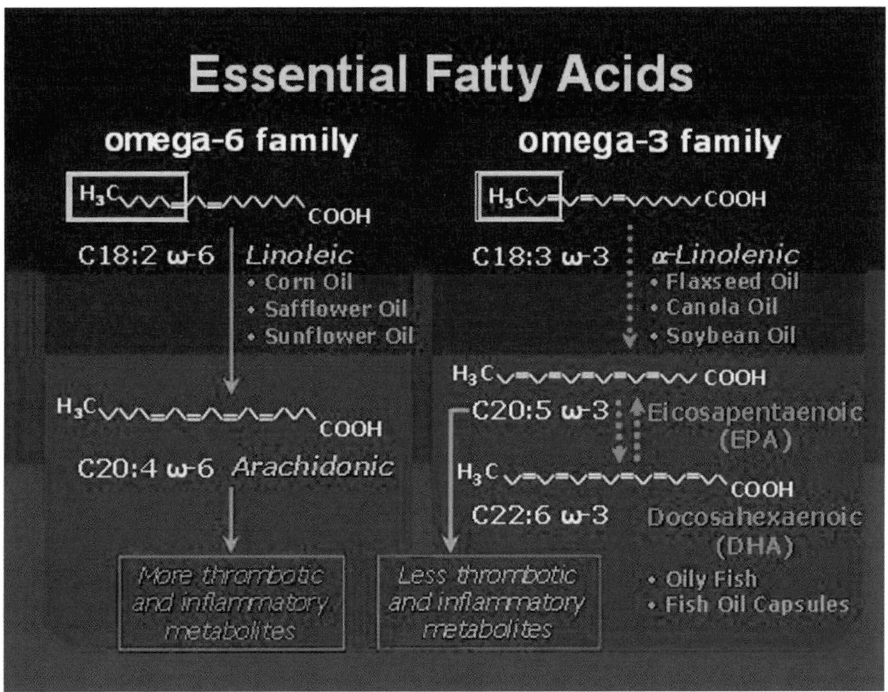

Recommendations for a healthy diet in non-pregnant or nursing adults generally include eating fish twice a week. Fish oil supplements appear to contain almost no mercury. However, fish oil taken for many months may cause a deficiency of vitamin E, and therefore, vitamin E is often added to commercial fish oil products. Fish liver oil also contains small amounts of the fat-soluble vitamins A and D.

Bad Fats

Too much of certain types of fats, such as saturated fats or *trans* fats, can increase blood cholesterol levels and the risk of coronary artery disease.

Saturated fats are usually solid or waxy at room temperature. They are found in red meat, high-fat dairy products (butter, cheese, whole milk, and ice cream), poultry skin, and egg yolks.

Some plant foods are also high in saturated fats (for example, coconut, coconut oil, palm oil, and palm kernel oil).

Trans fatty acids, or "*trans* fats," are produced by heating liquid vegetable oils in the presence of hydrogen, a process called hydrogenation. Since *trans* fats are more solid than oil, they are less likely to spoil. The more hydrogenated an oil is, the harder it will be at room temperature. For example, a tub of spread margarine is less hydrogenated and has fewer *trans* fats than stick margarine. Most of the *trans* fats in the American diet are found in commercially prepared baked goods, tub and stick margarines, snack foods, and processed foods. Commercially prepared fried foods, like french fries and onion rings, also may contain *trans* fats. Using *trans* fats in the manufacturing of foods keeps them fresh longer ("longer shelf life") and creates a less greasy texture.

Impact of Dietary Fats on Heart Disease

The classic diet-heart connection related the intake of saturated fats and cholesterol to the risk of coronary heart disease (CHD). More than twenty scientific studies now address diet and the risk of CHD. Higher cholesterol levels show a strong and consistent relationship with the incidence of CHD. The type of fat consumed appears to be more important than the amount of total fat. *Trans* fats increase the risk of CHD, while MUFA and PUFA decrease the risk.

Results from 49,000 women studied in a very important clinical research study, called the "Women's Health Initiative Dietary Modification Trial," showed that eating a low-fat diet for eight years did not prevent CHD, breast cancer, or colon cancer, and furthermore, was not associated with any weight loss. This unexpected result may be explained as follows: during a low-fat diet, carbohydrates are often used to replace fats, and include starchy foods such as pasta, white rice, and bread. Another problem is that a typical low-fat diet may avoid the intake of healthy or good fats. There is consistent scientific evidence that a high intake of either MUFA or PUFA lowers the risk for CHD. In the "Nurses' Health Study," the risk for CHD was decreased by about 30 to 40 percent by replacing 80 calories of carbohydrates with 80 calories of MUFA and/or PUFA.

It is well known that high blood LDL-cholesterol levels are associated with an increased risk for CHD. However, many research studies have shown that there is only a weak relationship between the amount of cholesterol eaten and the actual blood cholesterol levels or risk for CHD. The cholesterol content of the diet may still be important, but it is the cholesterol level in the bloodstream that ultimately is most important for health risks. For some people with high cholesterol, reducing the amount of cholesterol in the diet can have an impact on lowering blood cholesterol. For others, the amount of cholesterol eaten may have little impact on the circulating blood cholesterol level. In yet another study of over 80,000 female nurses, Harvard researchers actually found that increasing cholesterol intake by 200 milligrams for every 1,000 calories in the diet (about an egg a day) did not significantly increase the risk for CHD.

The liver is responsible for making 75 percent of blood cholesterol, while only 25 percent is absorbed from food. The biggest influence of the diet on the blood cholesterol is the type and combination of fats that are consumed. For instance, dietary saturated fats raise total blood cholesterol levels more than dietary cholesterol because saturated fats increase both HDL-cholesterol and LDL-cholesterol. However, the net effect is bad. This means that it is important to limit saturated fats in the diet. Simply put, the key to this healthy eating strategy is to substitute good fats for bad fats in the diet.

High consumption of *trans* fats, found mainly in partially hydrogenated vegetable oils and widely used by the food industry, has also been linked to an increased risk of CHD. *Trans* fat dietary intake has been substantially reduced in Europe compared to the US, although some US cities (such as New York and Philadelphia) have passed legislation eliminating *trans* fat use in restaurants.

Eating large amounts of high-fat foods adds excess calories and, when eaten on a regular basis, can lead to weight gain and obesity. Obesity is a risk factor for CHD, among other diseases, such as diabetes, cancer, gallstones, sleep apnea, and osteoarthritis.

DIETARY FATS			
FAT TYPE	**FOOD SOURCES**	**FORM AT ROOM TEMPERATURE**	**EFFECT ON BLOOD LIPIDS AND CHD RISK**
Mono-unsaturated	**Olives, olive oil, canola oil, peanut oil, cashews, almonds, peanuts and most other nuts, avocados**	**Liquid**	**Lowers LDL Raises HDL Lowers CHD risk**
Poly-unsaturated	**Corn, soybean, safflower, cottonseed oils, fish**	**Liquid**	**Lowers LDL Raises HDL Lowers CHD risk**
Saturated	**Whole milk, butter, solid shortening, lard, fatback, cheese, ice cream, red meat, chocolate, coconuts, coconut milk, coconut oil**	**Solid**	**Raises both LDL and HDL Raises CHD risk**
***Trans* Fats**	**Most margarines, vegetable shortening, partially hydrogenated vegetable oil, deep-fried chips, many fast foods, most baked goods**	**Solid or semi-solid**	**Raises LDL Raises CHD risk**

TYPE OF FAT	RECOMMENDATION
Total fats	Less than 35 % of total daily calories
Saturated fats	Less than 10 % of total daily calories
Dietary cholesterol	Less than 300 milligrams a day

The US Department of Agriculture (USDA) and the Department of Health and Human Services (HHS) have recommended upper limit values for saturated fats (less than 10% of daily calories) and dietary cholesterol (less than 300 mg a day) for healthy adults. Fat should make up no more than 35 percent of total daily calories. This means an 1,800-calorie diet should contain no more than 70 grams of fat (multiply 1,800 total daily calories by 35% (0.35) = 630 fat calories; then divide 630 calories by 9 calories/gram of fat = 70 grams of daily fat). Remember, this is an upper daily limit for fat calories, and most of these fat calories should come from dietary MUFA and PUFA sources.

Eating fish may help prevent heart disease in several ways. First, dietary fish replaces red meat or other less-healthy sources of protein in the diet. Second, omega-3 fats in fish can lower serum triglyceride levels. Third, fish appears to protect the heart from developing disturbances in the heartbeat rhythm (see figure 2).

Both farmed fish and fresh fish appear to have the same amount of omega-3 fatty acid (eicosapentaenoic acid [EPA] + docosahexaenoic acid [DHA]) content. There is strong evidence from human research trials that omega-3 fatty acids from fish or fish oil supplements (EPA + DHA) significantly reduce blood triglyceride levels. These benefits appear to vary directly with the dose used: low doses cause small effects, and high doses cause large effects. The smallest effects can occur with doses as low as 2 grams each day of omega-3 fatty acids. Larger effects, which lower triglyceride levels by 25 to 40 percent, can occur with doses of 4 grams each day. These beneficial effects of omega-3 fats, or fish oils, may actually increase the beneficial effects of the "statin" drugs. Statins inhibit the function of an enzyme called "HMG-CoA reductase," which helps control cholesterol production in the body. The effects of fish oil on high triglyceride levels are similar in patients with or without diabetes, and also in those patients with kidney disease who are receiving dialysis.

A physician should be consulted prior to the use of omega-3 fatty acids. This is because dietary supplements can have adverse effects. With omega-3 fat doses greater than 3 grams each day, there is an increased risk of bleeding. Omega-3 fatty acid use may increase HDL-cholesterol by 1 to 3 percent, but may also increase LDL-cholesterol by 5 to 10 percent. Thus, omega-3 fatty acid use will not be of significant benefit for total or LDL-cholesterol lowering.

Impact of Dietary Fats on Diabetes and Obesity

Presently, about two-thirds of the US population is at least overweight (BMI greater than 25) and about half of these people are obese (BMI greater than 30). Counting calories and fat grams is a well-recognized means of weight loss and was the strategy selected for achieving weight reduction for two important clinical research studies: the Diabetes Prevention Program (DPP) and Look AHEAD trials. Participants in these studies were educated on calorie and fat gram counting and given reference booklets. Recommended calorie and fat gram dietary intake was based on initial body weight. The diets provided 25 to 30 percent of calories from fat and less than 10 percent total fat as saturated fat. Calorie and fat gram targets were selected to promote one to two pounds per week weight loss. In the DPP trial, changing diet and exercise habits resulted in modest weight loss in obese men and women who had pre-diabetes. The results of the Look AHEAD trial will be available in 2012.

POPULATION	AHA RECOMMENDATION FOR OMEGA-3 FATTY ACID INTAKE
Patients without documented CHD	Eat a variety of fish (preferably oily fish) at least twice weekly. Include oils and foods rich in alpha-linolenic acid (flaxseed, canola and soybean oils; and walnuts)
Patients with documented CHD	Consume ~1 gram/day EPA+DHA (preferably oily fish). EPA+DHA supplements could be considered in consultation with a physician.
Patients needing triglyceride lowering	2-4 grams/day EPA+DHA provided as capsules under a physician's care.

SOURCE	1 GRAM EPA+DHA EQUIVALENT
Fish	2-3 ounces/day oily fish (salmon, sardines, mackerel)
Cod Liver Oil	1 tsp
Dietary Supplements	*Low potency* (drug stores): ~300 mg EPA+DHA per gram (requires ~3 grams fish oil) *Mid potency* (mail order): 500-700 mg EPA+DHA per gram (requires ~2 grams fish oil) *High potency* (Rx): ~850 mg EPA+DHA per gram (requires ~1 gram omega-3 acid ethyl esters)

High-fiber diets may in part protect against diabetes, obesity, and CHD by lowering insulin levels and improving insulin resistance. The beneficial effect of increased fiber intake on insulin levels, weight gain, and other CHD risk factors is stronger than the effect of decreased total or saturated fat intake. A high-fiber diet, compared to a low-fiber diet, is associated with a 40 to 50 percent reduction in the risk of CHD and stroke. For each 10 grams a day of fiber intake, there is a 14 percent less chance for having a heart attack or related problem. This risk reduction was greater with intake of fiber from cereals and fruits than with fiber from vegetables.

Suggested Readings

American Diabetes Association. "Specific types of fat." http://www.diabetes.org/nutrition-and-recipes/nutrition/foodlabel/specific-fats.jsp (accessed on October 12, 2008).

Harvard School of Public Health. "The Nutrition Source: Knowledge for healthy eating." http://www.hsph.harvard.edu/nutritionsource/index.html (accessed on October 12, 2008).

MayoClinic.com. "Healthy Living." http://mayoclinic.com/health/HealthyLivingIndex/HealthyLivingIndex/ (accessed on October 12, 2008).

Faqs.org. "Nutrition and well-being A to Z: Fats" http://www.faqs.org/nutrition/Erg-Foo/Fats.html (accessed on October 12, 2008).

US Food and Drug Administration. "Questions and answers about trans fat nutrition labeling." http://www.foodsafety.gov/~dms/qatrans2.html (accessed on October 12, 2008).

Chapter 2.3

Protein

Jason M. Hollander, MD, CNSP

Protein Function

The word *protein* is derived from the Greek word *prota,* which means "of primary importance," emphasizing the importance of protein in the human diet. Unlike carbohydrates and fats, our bodies cannot store protein for future use. All proteins are in a state of constant turnover; they are broken down into building blocks known as amino acids and rebuilt to meet the many needs of the human body.

Proteins make up important structural elements in our bodies including cartilage, ligaments, and the keratin in our nails and hair. Other structural proteins are "motor" proteins that form muscles and allow us to move about. Certain proteins carry information from one cell to another. Other proteins receive this information and then aid in processing the message. Enzymes are proteins that make chemical reactions work. Finally, there are other important chemicals in the body that are not actually proteins, but require the nitrogen component of protein. Examples of these chemicals are nucleic acids (found in DNA), certain hormones, and some neurotransmitters, which are important for brain function.

Protein Structure

Proteins are comprised of small molecules known as amino acids (See figure, page 48). There are twenty important amino acids that are incorporated into proteins. The most important feature of an amino acid is the ability to form a special chemical bond, called a "peptide bond," with other amino acids. A chain of two to twenty amino acids is called an "oligopeptide." If the chain of amino acids is even longer, then it is called a "polypeptide," which contains from twenty to several thousand amino acids. Polypeptide chains twist and bend in unique ways based on complicated chemical principles to form proteins. The ultimate order and shape of joined amino acids determines the structure and function of each unique protein.

Amino acids are generated in the body in three different ways:

- They enter our bodies as protein in the food we eat.
- They are made in our bodies.
- They come from the breakdown of protein already in body tissue.

Free amino acids exist as individual molecules that are not part of a larger peptide or protein structure. Free amino acids are shuttled through the bloodstream to areas in the body where they are needed. The body then uses these free amino acids to assemble new proteins. Amino acids can also be burned as fuel when their supply is in excess of bodily requirements. Finally, individual amino acids can be turned into related molecules, like serotonin, epinephrine, and histamine, that convey information within the body.

While it is clear that protein is an important part of our diet, the metabolism of amino acids generates a nitrogen-containing compound known as ammonia, which is toxic at high levels. The liver converts ammonia to urea by a number of reactions known as the "urea cycle." Urea is a molecule essentially containing two ammonia molecules. The kidneys can then more safely excrete urea. Therefore, diets high in protein necessitate the consumption of large amounts of water to ensure that urea can leave the body safely.

Protein Types

Before protein requirements can be discussed, one must understand that from a nutritional standpoint, the most important distinction among amino acids is the distinction between those that are "essential" and those that are "nonessential." Essential amino acids are those that are not made in sufficient quantities in the body to prevent a disease and must be provided in food. We must consume a minimum amount of essential amino acids in our diet in order to maintain a healthy state. Examples of essential amino acids include:

- the "metabolically indispensable" amino acids threonine and lysine;
- the "branched-chain" amino acids: leucine, isoleucine, and valine;
- tryptophan, phenylalanine, methionine; and
- for infants and growing children: cysteine, tyrosine, histidine, and arginine.

"Conditionally essential" amino acids are not made in sufficient quantities for the metabolic needs of the body during certain forms of stress. These include arginine, cysteine, glutamine, histidine, proline, serine, and tyrosine. The remaining amino acids found in the body are called "nonessential" or "metabolically dispensable" and can easily be formed from other amino acids even if they are not part of the diet.

Protein Requirements

In general, protein must be consumed in a quantity that is sufficient to meet a body's metabolic demands. In other words, one must consume enough protein to provide amino acids for all of the pathways discussed above. For example, during times of growth, illness, pregnancy, and lactation, protein requirements are increased. Calculating the nutritional protein requirements would seem quite possible, but in fact, these calculations are very difficult. Proteins are constantly being broken down and then rebuilt again. Moreover, many different amino acids can be made by the body. Through a process called "adaptation," the body can conserve protein when necessary, like during starvation, by burning fewer calories for energy and recycling more metabolic fuels.

Protein can even be salvaged from urea. Therefore, the body can adapt to various levels of protein intake.

The process of adaptation clearly makes defining a Recommended Dietary Allowance (RDA; the dietary intake level that is sufficient to meet the requirements of 97 to 98 percent of the population) very difficult. Currently, the RDA for protein for an adult male is 56 grams per day. The RDA for an adult female is 46 grams per day. The typical American diet provides protein well in excess of the RDAs.

Protein Sources in the Diet

Protein can be found in a variety of foods from both plant and animal origin. Protein derived from animal sources, like meat, poultry, fish, eggs, milk, cheese, and yogurt, provides all of the essential amino acids and are considered "complete" proteins. Proteins derived from plant sources, like legumes, nuts, grains, vegetables, and seeds, are typically deficient in one or more of the essential amino acids and are called "incomplete" proteins. Healthy sources of high biological value protein (see below) are, therefore, egg whites, lean meats, low-fat or no-fat dairy products, and legumes (beans).

To complicate the discussion, not all protein-containing foods are digested and absorbed to the same degree. This is a concept known as "digestibility." Animal products typically have very high digestibility scores, while other sources of protein are variably digested. The degree to which protein is absorbed from food and incorporated into one's body can be quantified and is called "biological value" (BV). By convention, BV is often given as the percentage utilization compared to a reference protein of high digestibility, commonly an egg. An egg is assigned a value of 100 percent with other sources of protein receiving lesser values. A list of common sources of protein and select BVs is provided in table 1.

Protein Deficiency

In developed countries, protein deficiency is rare. However, protein deficiency does occur, and when it does, it is usually the result of one of the following:

- Unusual dietary habits
- Inability to absorb protein in the gastrointestinal tract due to certain illnesses
- Excessive protein loss from either the kidneys or the gastrointestinal tract
- Abnormal protein metabolism due to certain diseases and hormonal disorders
- Increased protein turnover and breakdown due to a severe injury, burn, infection, or chronic disease

In these instances, the delivery of extra protein is necessary to sustain life and promote healing. Without adequate supply, the body must break down tissues to provide amino acids for vital functions. Left unchecked, this process leads to severe weakness, disability, and ultimately death.

Food	Amount	Protein (grams)	Biological Value (BV)
Egg	1 (medium)	6	100
Beans	8 oz.	8	96
Milk	8oz.	8	60 - 91
Cheese	1oz.	7	84
Beef	3 oz.	24	69 - 80
Chicken	3 oz.	27	79
Fish	3oz.	23	70 - 76
Tofu	½ cup	10	47 – 64
Rice, Brown	1 cup	4.5	57
Peanuts	½ cup	19	55

BodyBuildingPro.com. www.bodybuildingpro.com/proteinrating.html (accessed on September 22, 2008).

Hoffman JR, Falvo MJ. Protein – Which is best? J Sport Med Nutr 2004; 3: 118–130.

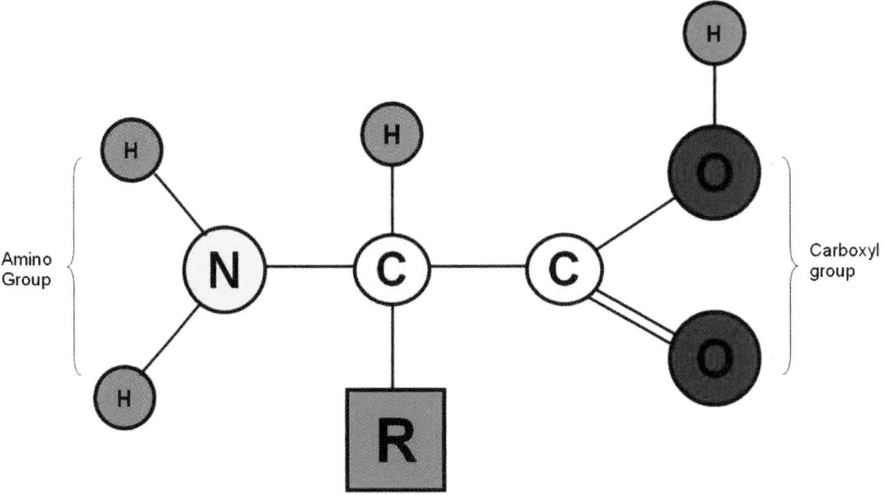

Each amino acid is made up of an amino group, a carboxyl group, and a unique side chain, R, attached to a central carbon (See text, page 49)

Suggested Reading

Centers for Disease Control and Prevention. "Nutrition for everyone." http://www.cdc.gov/nccdphp/dnpa/nutrition/nutrition_for_everyone/basics/protein.htm (accessed on September 22, 2008).

Harvard School of Public Health. "The Nutrition Source: Protein." www.hsph.harvard.edu/nutritionsource/what-should-you-eat/protein/ (accessed on September 22, 2008).

KidsHealth. "Learning about proteins." http://kidshealth.org/kid/nutrition/food/protein.html (accessed on September 22, 2008).

Rinzler CA. *Nutrition for Dummies, 4th Edition.* Wiley Publishing, Inc., Hoboken, NJ, 2006.

Sizer F, Whitney E. *Nutrition: Concepts and Controversies 11th Edition.* Thomson Wadsworth, Belmont, CA.2005.

Chapter 2.4

Vitamins

Martin M. Grajower, MD, FACP, FACE

Vitamins are defined as chemical substances that cannot be made in sufficient amounts by the body, yet are important for normal functioning of the body. We rely on the food we eat to get most of our vitamins. In general, vitamins are found in small amounts in different foods. Most of the functions of our bodies depend on vitamins to work normally.

For example, vitamin A is critical for normal vision, and without it, a person can have difficulty with vision, especially at night. We need vitamin D to grow normally and to maintain our bones in good health so they do not break easily. Vitamin E helps us fight off damage to our blood vessels from harmful chemicals found in foods we eat. Vitamin K is important for normal blood clotting; low levels of vitamin K make it harder to stop bleeding if one is cut or injured. Vitamin B12 helps us maintain healthy nerves; without it, we can become confused, forgetful, or lose our balance.

Pregnant women need extra vitamins because the growing fetus relies on the mother to provide it with the vitamins it needs to develop normally. Certain vitamins like folic acid are important right from the beginning of pregnancy. For this reason, doctors recommend that pregnant women take extra folic acid, either as part of their "prenatal" multivitamin or as a separate folic acid tablet. Many women will begin taking these vitamins even before they get pregnant, just to be safe.

While vitamins are essential for good health, too much of a good thing is not good. Many vitamins can cause problems if we get too much. While it is rare to have too much of any one vitamin from eating food, since there is so little in food, it is possible to get too much from taking over-the-counter vitamins. The table below lists some of the problems that can develop from too much of any one vitamin.

Vitamin	Sources: how we get it naturally	Function: why we need it	Deficiency: what happens if we don't have enough	Toxicity: what happens if we get too much of the vitamin
A	fish, liver oils, liver, egg yolk, butter, cream, vitamin-A fortified margarine, dark leafy vegetables, yellow fruits, red palm oil	Cells of the eye that see, healthy skin	Difficulty seeing at night, bad skin	Headache, peeling of skin, swollen liver, abnormal bones
D	Ultraviolet radiation of the skin from the sun, fortified milk, fish liver oils, butter, egg yolk, liver	To absorb calcium and phosphorus from food we eat and to develop healthy bones	Abnormal & weak bones which are more likely to break	Loss of appetite, kidneys stop working, abnormal calcium deposits in different parts of the body
E	Vegetable oil, wheat germ, leafy vegetables, egg yolk, margarine, beans	Protects cells from damage by bad chemicals in the body	Damage to red blood cells, nerves, and muscles	Interfere with the normal function of many cells in different parts of the body
K	Leafy vegetables, pork, liver, vegetable oils	To form chemicals necessary to form clots that stop bleeding	Abnormal & excessive bleeding	

People who eat a normal diet, including vegetables, fruit, dairy, and protein (meat, cheese, and eggs), will rarely be lacking in vitamins, with the notable exception of vitamin D. Therefore, these people do not need to take any vitamin supplements. On the other hand, people who do not eat a balanced diet or people who eat very little (like some old or sick people) may need to take a "one-a-day" multivitamin pill. In addition, some people may need to take specific vitamin supplements for individual reasons. Generally, these people will be told to do so by their doctor based on a blood test. For example, some people cannot absorb certain vitamins like B12; therefore, they may need to get B12 injections from their doctors.

Over the past few years, research studies have shown that the majority of women over the age of fifty, and many men, are lacking in vitamin D. The likely reason has to do with not enough exposure to sunlight and the use of sunscreens (important for the prevention of skin cancer), together with a diet low in dairy products, especially milk. For this reason, most women over the age of fifty would likely benefit from a vitamin D supplement. A simple blood test by the doctor can tell if a person is getting enough vitamin D or needs to take more.

Suggested Readings

Center for Nutrition Policy and Promotion, US Department of Agriculture. "Dietary Guidelines for Americans 2005." www.healthierus.gov/dietaryguidelines (accessed on October 18, 2008).

Harvard School of Public Health. "The Nutrition Source: Vitamins." http://www.hsph.harvard.edu/nutritionsource/what-should-you-eat/vitamins/ (accessed on September 21, 2008).

Northwestern University. "NorthwesternNutrition: Vitamins." http://www.feinberg.northwestern.edu/nutrition/factsheets/vitamins.html (accessed on September 21, 2008).

Rinzler CA. *Nutrition for Dummies, 4th Edition.* Wiley Publishing, Inc., Hoboken NJ, 2006.

U.S. National Library of Medicine and the National Institutes of Health. "Medline Plus: Vitamins." http://www.nlm.nih.gov/medlineplus/vitamins.html (accessed on September 21, 2008).

Chapter 2.5

Minerals

Arthur Chausmer, MD

What are Minerals?

We need minerals for many reasons, some to maintain the structure of certain chemicals and some to maintain the function of certain chemicals (see table 1). In the medical world, the term *mineral* is used to describe naturally occurring nutrients that are not "organic," meaning that they do not contain the element carbon. Examples of such minerals are sodium, iron, potassium, and calcium, which have a positive charge, and iodine and fluorine, which have a negative charge.

The diet is the only source for minerals. Unlike many proteins or other substances, the body cannot make or destroy minerals, only absorb them, use them, or excrete them. In terms of use, most minerals are used to force other molecules, usually proteins such as enzymes or hormones, into the right shape so they can attach to other things and do what they are supposed to do. Zinc and copper hold many proteins in a shape that allows them to bind with cell membranes and exert their action. Having a certain shape is like becoming a key that interacts with other molecules, which are locks. Enzymes are proteins that can require minerals to interact with other chemicals in order to make certain reactions happen.

Other minerals hold parts of larger molecules together. Iron holds together the four rings of hemoglobin. Cobalt holds together the structure of vitamin B12. Some other minerals regulate the ability of cell membranes to transport substances, like glucose, from the blood to the inside of the cell. Still other minerals maintain the structure of membranes. Sodium and potassium have important functions in this way.

Many minerals can perform several functions in different tissues. For example, calcium and phosphorus are the major substances in the formation of bone. However, calcium also acts inside cells to regulate the contraction of muscles or secretion of hormones. Also, phosphorus is important for the utilization of food energy within a cell. There is generally more than one function for minerals.

Sodium

Sodium (represented by the chemical symbol "Na") is present in almost everything we eat, usually in the form of salt, which is sodium chloride. The body has very complex mechanisms for regulating the concentration of sodium in the blood and extracellular fluids. It is very important for the concentration of sodium to be closely regulated and kept within a very narrow range for healthy body function.

One important function of sodium is to maintain the proper pressure of fluids in the body, called "osmotic pressure." This helps with blood pressure and the volume of our cells, which are mostly composed of water. In many people, an increased amount of sodium in the diet can worsen high blood pressure, which can result in heart disease, kidney disease, or stroke. This effect of sodium is particularly important since the average American diet is high in salt. Several of the medications used to treat high blood pressure act by increasing the loss of sodium through the kidney. High salt intake while taking these medications to reduce blood pressure makes them much less effective.

Since there are many effective mechanisms for regulating blood sodium concentrations, high blood sodium is rare and usually caused by too little water intake, leading to "dehydration." It is hard to have a diet low enough in salt to cause medical problems. Almost always, problems with low blood sodium concentrations are caused by too much water rather than too little sodium. When low sodium is not the result of too much water, it is almost always caused by some other serious medical condition or medications, and not by diet.

Potassium

Frequently, sodium and potassium (represented by the chemical symbol "K") act as checks and balances for each other. For instance, the fluid outside the cell is high in sodium and relatively low in potassium, while the fluid inside the cell is high in potassium and relatively low in sodium. This balance must be maintained for all cells to function.

As with sodium, it is hard to have high or low blood concentrations of potassium based on diet alone. Again, this is because there are very effective body mechanisms to keep potassium levels in a narrow range. Low potassium levels can occur though with the use of "diuretics" or "water pills" used to control high blood pressure. In addition to increasing salt and water losses from the body with increased urination, there are also increased potassium losses. This can lead to low blood potassium levels, which is easily treated with potassium supplements.

Calcium

Calcium (represented by the chemical symbol "Ca") is necessary for many body functions and, along with phosphorus, is the major component of bone. Calcium is also essential for many of the basic functions in all of the cells of the body, particularly nerve and muscle function. If there is too little calcium in these cells, they can become hypersensitive. Muscles can start to twitch, contract, and then go into spasm, and nerves can become hyperactive and cause seizures. Too much calcium in the blood can have the opposite effect, resulting in the muscles and nerves not being able to contract or function. If the blood calcium gets too high, coma and death can occur. Long-term lack of adequate calcium can result in bone loss.

The body has different ways to regulate calcium. Vitamin D is essential for the body to absorb calcium from the diet. Most of our vitamin D is made in the skin from cholesterol. This vitamin D is not active and has to be transported in the blood to the liver, where it is made into 25-hydroxyvitamin D. This chemical is then transported to the kidney to be made into 1,25-dihydroxyvitamin D, which is the form that actually increases calcium absorption. If there is too little sun exposure, liver disease, or kidney disease, then calcium absorption is not enough. Fortunately, we can also get vitamin D from our food, such as in fortified milk and certain fish, or by taking vitamin D-containing supplements. In general, we should probably have about 800 units of vitamin D a day in our diets if we do not get a lot of sun exposure. Too much vitamin D can be toxic, so more is not necessarily better without having a doctor watch for problems.

As adults, we should also have about 1,000-1,200 milligrams of calcium a day in our diets, depending on age and gender. People who do not get much calcium from their diets may benefit from calcium supplements, again after consulting with a doctor, since some people need more and others may need less. Dairy foods, certain nuts and seeds, soy products, some vegetables, beans, and some fish are good sources of calcium.

Magnesium

Magnesium (represented by the chemical symbol "Mg") is present in all cells and is essential for proper cell function at virtually every level. It is the fourth most abundant mineral in the body. It is a cofactor for a wide variety of cell functions, such as immune function and glucose metabolism. Magnesium also allows the vascular system to maintain a normal blood pressure. Low magnesium is usually a result of very poor dietary intake, such as is seen in alcoholics or malabsorptive conditions. Lack of magnesium prevents many of the mechanisms that act to keep cell and blood calcium in the normal range. As a result, one of the major effects of a low magnesium level is a low blood calcium level, which can result in "tetany" (uncontrollable muscle contractions), seizures, and heart irregularities. In plants, magnesium acts as a center for chlorophyll, much like iron acts as a center for hemoglobin. As a result, green leafy vegetables and seafood are excellent sources of magnesium.

Iodine

Dietary iodine (represented by the chemical symbol "I") deficiency used to be common and resulted in goiter, which is an enlarged thyroid gland. The thyroid gland makes hormones that regulate the activity of all of the cells in the body. These hormones, thyroxine and triiodothyronine, sometimes called "T4" and "T3," respectively, contain iodine as an essential part of their structure. Thyroxine contains four molecules of iodine, and triiodothyronine contains three molecules of iodine.

Goiter used to be very common in the United States, particularly in the central plains where there was little access to seafood and the soil was very poor in iodine. By government regulation, iodine was added to virtually all table salt, and white bread was enriched with, among other things, iodine. As a result, dietary iodine deficiency is virtually unknown in the United States except among populations that have very restrictive dietary requirements.

Iron

Iron (represented by the chemical symbol "Fe") functions in the hemoglobin molecule that carries oxygen in the red blood cells throughout the body. Hemoglobin consists of four ring-like molecules, which are held together by the iron molecule. Maintaining the structure of hemoglobin is the only significant role for iron. Many foods have a lot of iron, particularly meats and green leafy vegetables.

Inadequate amounts of iron in the diet can result in the common form of iron deficiency anemia. Iron deficiency anemia is defined as a decreased number and size of red blood cells. Most of the iron lost from the body is in the form of small amounts of intestinal cells and blood in the stool and, to a much greater extent, in the blood loss that occurs with menstruation in women. As a result of this blood loss, postpubertal girls and premenopausal women are at a much greater risk of iron deficiency anemia and frequently need supplemental iron. This is rather easy for a doctor to diagnose.

Excess iron in the body is relatively rare and is generally the result of problems with the blood-forming systems. Nevertheless, excessive iron intake, typically as a result of iron supplements, can result in iron overload since there are few mechanisms by which the body can rid itself of excess iron. "Hemochromatosis" is an inherited disorder of iron overload that can affect the liver, heart, pituitary gland, and many other organs.

Trace Elements

Trace elements include zinc (Zn), copper (Cu), selenium (Se), manganese (Mn), nickel (Ni), and chromium (Cr). These are required in very small amounts, which is why they are called trace elements. Zinc and copper are used in virtually all cells as structural parts of enzymes. Chromium has been shown to be necessary for normal glucose metabolism, although the exact mechanisms have not been completely explained. As with most other minerals, these trace elements are found in many foods, including vegetables and nuts and meats.

How much is enough?

It is important to note that with many of these minerals, claims have been made that we do not get enough of them for good health, although evidence of dietary deficiency states is very uncommon in people who do not have some other, underlying, medical problem. While we clearly need enough, it is not clear that more than enough is better. At the present time, the ranges of intake suggested by the Recommended Dietary Allowances appear to be the best guide to good nutrition. For those for whom there is some question about whether the diet is adequate, one reputable multivitamin tablet with minerals may be a good insurance policy. There is no evidence that more than one tablet a day has any health benefit for those without special needs. As one might expect, those people with special needs should be under the care of a knowledgeable physician.

The RDA, or Recommended Dietary Allowance, was developed during the Second World War and represents estimates for a young male population. These estimates are being updated in stages and currently represented as "Dietary Reference Intakes," or "DRI" (see appendix 6.1). There are, of course, differences between males and females and for different ages. While one size does not fit all and there is some evidence that these numbers may not be optimal, they do provide a good general guideline for total daily dietary intake, not supplemental intake, for these selected minerals. They are presented here only as examples and rough guidelines (see table 2). This table should not be considered definitive for any individual.

Mineral	Function	Deficiency signs	Toxicities
Sodium	Maintains blood volume	Seizures	Seizures, hypertension
Potassium	Stabilize cell membranes	Heart rhythm problems	Heart rhythm problems
Calcium	Bone structure, muscle and nerve activity	Muscle twitches, severe muscle contraction osteoporosis	Weakness, coma, heart rhythm problems
Magnesium	Regulates metabolism within cells	Low serum calcium, seizures	Coma, heart rhythm problems
Iron	Central part of hemoglobin	Anemia	Multi organ failure
Zinc	Holds enzymes in proper structure	Loss of taste and smell, dwarfism, male hypogonadism	Flu like syndrome lasting several days.
Iodine	Active part of thyroid hormones	Goiter, low thyroid function	Can block or stimulate thyroid activity outside of normal range
Copper	Holds enzymes in proper structures	Neurologic abnormalities	Liver malfunction
Chlorine	Couples with sodium, regulates membranes	Makes the body less acid which makes some enzymes not work optimally	Makes the body more acid which makes some enzymes not work optimally.
Phosphorus	Combines with Ca to make bone, regulates energy production within cells	Muscle failure	Calcium phosphate deposits in tissues and skin

Table 1. Function, deficiency states, and toxicities of some common minerals

Mineral	Lower limit	Upper limit
Calcium (Ca)	1200 milligrams	2500 milligrams
Potassium (K)	700 milligrams	n/a
Magnesium (Mg)	400 milligrams	n/a
Iron (Fe)	8 milligrams	45 milligrams
Copper (Cu)	900 micrograms	10000 micrograms
Zinc (Zn)	11 micrograms	40 micrograms
Chromium (Cr)	35 micrograms	n/a
Iodine	150 micrograms	1100 micrograms
Selenium (Se)	55 micrograms	400 micrograms
Manganese (Mn)	7 milligrams	11 milligrams

Table 2. Upper and lower limit values for daily mineral ingestion

Suggested Readings

Center for Nutrition Policy and Promotion, US Department of Agriculture. "Dietary Guidelines for Americans 2005." www.healthierus.gov/dietaryguidelines (accessed on October 18, 2008).

Northwestern University. "NorthwesterNutrition: Minerals." http://www.feinberg.northwestern.edu/nutrition/factsheets/minerals.html (accessed on September 1, 2008).

Rinzler CA. *Nutrition for Dummies, 4th Edition.* Wiley Publishing, Inc., Hoboken, NJ, 2006.

Chapter 2.6

Some Really Healthy Foods

Jeffrey I. Mechanick, MD, FACP, FACE, FACN
Elise M. Brett, MD, FACE, CNSP

There are very few absolute "good" or "bad" foods when taken in the context of a healthy eating program and healthy lifestyle. Rather, there are certain foods that represent healthier choices than other foods. Bearing in mind that our definition of nutrition is the interaction of our diet with our metabolism, what is healthy for one person may not be healthy for another. Nevertheless, there are some foods that are generally considered healthy for "most" people, and some of these will be listed and discussed in this chapter. Following the discussion of each food will be a table of important nutrients found in the food discussed. There may also be a section and table providing other foods that are comparable. Obviously, this is not a complete list, but it can provide some insight about what constitutes a "healthy food." This chapter can also prepare you to include healthy foods in a healthy meal. By regularly eating healthy meals, you are on your way to a healthy lifestyle.

You may have heard the terms *functional foods, superfoods,* and/or *superfruits.* These are terms that have been created, primarily for commercial or marketing purposes, to indicate that these natural foods contain special health-promoting chemicals. Since all natural foods have some nutritional benefit, these terms are not particularly helpful and are not referred to in this chapter.

The following list of Power of Prevention Healthy Foods is presented in alphabetical order. Important attributes of healthy foods are given below, but not every food will have every attribute; that is, not every healthy food is "perfect":

- High fiber
- High phytochemical (plant-derived chemicals that are thought to promote good health) content
- High biological value protein (high biological value protein means that a particular food contains all of the essential amino acids at a sufficient quantity for the portion size)
- Relatively high in "good" polyunsaturated (PUFA) or monounsaturated (MUFA) fatty acids
- Relatively low in calories
- Relatively low in saturated fats
- Low in added sugar
- "Whole" foods, which are not processed

Power of Prevention Healthy Food #1: ALMONDS

Almonds are one example of a healthy food that is enjoyed worldwide. Almonds are a rich dietary source of vitamin E and monounsaturated fatty acids (MUFA). Almonds are a staple in the Mediterranean diet, which is high in MUFA and associated with lipid-lowering properties and reduced risk for heart disease. The almond tree is native to the Middle East, although the state of California now produces much of the world's crop. Almonds may be eaten as a snack "raw," blanched, roasted, or toasted. Marcona almonds from Spain have a particularly smooth, softer texture and sweet taste and are often fried in olive oil. One culinary use of almonds is as a crunchy coating for fish or chicken ("almondine"). Almonds are also used in some Indian lamb dishes. Of course, almonds are a common ingredient in desserts such as cakes, cookies, pies, nougat and baklava. Almond butter is a popular alternative to peanut butter for those with peanut allergies. Almond flour is a low-carbohydrate alternative that may be beneficial for people with diabetes. One cup of almond flour has only 20 grams of carbohydrate, of which 10 grams is healthy fiber. Almond milk can be a nice soy-free alternative for those who are lactose-intolerant or vegan (a vegetarian who also avoids eggs and dairy products).

	Nutritional Information for Almonds:
Serving size	*1 ounce (28 grams) or 20-25 medium size nuts (dry-roasted, no salt added)*
Total calories	*167*
Protein (grams)	*6.2*
Fat (grams; type)	*14.8; MUFA 9.4 – PUFA 3.5*
Carbohydrate (grams)	*5.4*
Fiber (grams)	*3.3*
Other benefits	*Vitamin E 7.3 mg (36% daily needs) plenty of B-complex vitamins, arginine, magnesium, manganese and copper*
Comparisons	*one ounce of walnuts contains 183 calories, 18 grams of fat, 2 grams of fiber, plenty of B-complex vitamins but a higher ratio of PUFA 13.2 grams to MUFA 2.5 grams than almonds*

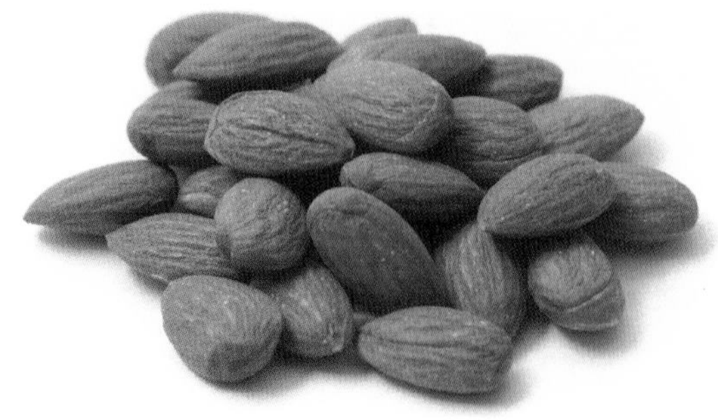

Power of Prevention Healthy Food #2: APPLE

Apples are one example of the many stimulating, nourishing, and healthy fruits that are available. Apples have a moderate amount of fiber and vitamins A and C with relatively few calories. Apples are also rich in phytochemicals such as polyphenols (including the flavonoid, quercetin) and triterpenoids (from the apple peel) which have antioxidant, anti-inflammatory and even anti-tumor properties. The apple is one of the world's most widely cultivated tree fruits, with the US being the second largest producer, behind China. There are hundreds of varieties of apples. Some are best for eating fresh while others are ideal for cooking or making juice. In short, apples are filling, very healthy, and serve as a great snack or dessert.

Nutritional Information for Apples:	
Serving size	*one medium apple with skin (3' diameter; 161 grams)*
Total calories	*94.6*
Protein (grams)	*0.5*
Fat (grams)	*0.3*
Carbohydrate (grams)	*25.1*
Fiber (grams)	*4.4*
Other benefits	*8.4 mg vitamin C (14% daily needs)* *98.3 units vitamin A (2% daily needs)* *5.5 mcg folate (1% daily needs)*
Comparisons	*50% of the fiber (2 grams) in the skin*

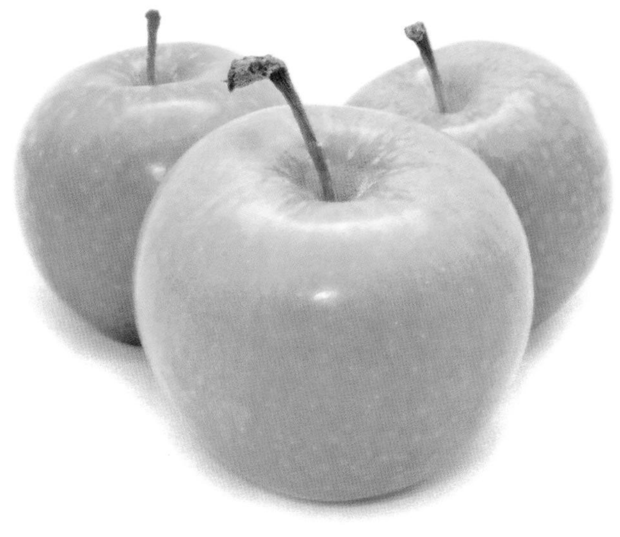

Power of Prevention Healthy Food #3: AVOCADO

The avocado is a fruit that contains lots of healthy fats like MUFA and polyunsaturated fatty acids (PUFA). Avocados are also rich in fiber, potassium, phosphorus, magnesium, zinc, and vitamins, particularly folic acid, vitamin C, vitamin B5 (pantothenic acid), and vitamin B6 (pyridoxine). Avocados are typically used for savory dishes such as salads, sandwiches, soups, sauces, salsas, and, of course, guacamole. Avocados grow on trees native to Mexico and South America; they were originally cultivated in pre-Incan times as long ago as 750 B.C. Now, the US (mainly Southern California) is the third largest producer behind Mexico and Indonesia. It should be noted that, while healthy, avocados are relatively high in calories.

Nutritional Information for Avocados:	
Serving size	*one average avocado*
Total calories	*322*
Protein (grams)	*4 (high biological quality)*
Fat (grams; type)	*29.5; MUFA 19.7 – PUFA 3.7*
Carbohydrate (grams)	*17.1*
Fiber (grams)	*13.5*
Other benefits	*vitamin K 42.2 mcg (53% daily needs)* *folate 163 mcg (41% daily needs)* *vitamin C 20.1 mg (33% daily needs)* *plenty of B-complex vitamins, potassium and copper*
Comparisons	*a California avocado is smaller (227 calories) with 21 grams of fat and 9 grams of fiber, compared with the larger Florida avocado (365 calories) that has 31 grams of fat and 17 grams of fiber*

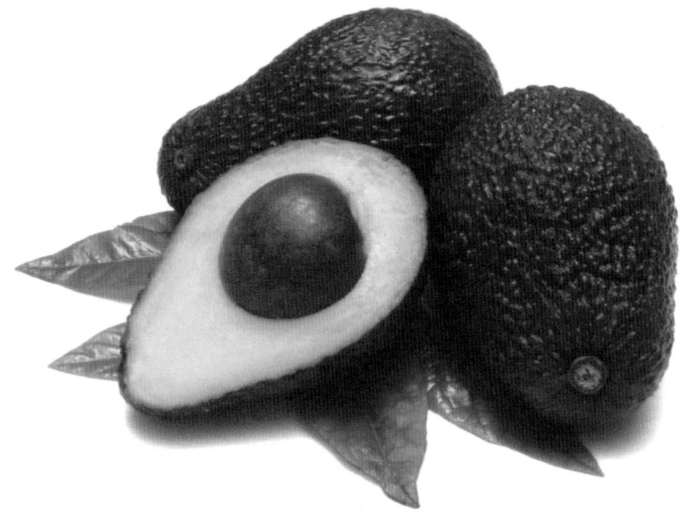

Power of Prevention Healthy Food #4: BEANS

Beans are an example of a healthy food: they are relatively low in calories, low in fat, and high in fiber, and have essential vitamins and minerals. Historically, beans were an excellent source of high biological value protein, especially when meat was scarce. Beans are an important component of vegan (no meat, eggs, or dairy) diets. Many beans (red and kidney beans) contain a harmful chemical called "phytohaemagglutinin," which is destroyed by boiling for a minimum of 10 minutes. Beans are associated with flatulence resulting from increased gas production in the intestines. This gas is produced by intestinal bacteria that digest certain types of sugar chemicals found in the fiber in the beans. This can be a problem in certain social situations, beans have a definite beneficial effect on "good" bacteria of the intestine and may reduce the risks of heart disease and some cancers because of their high fiber content. The navy bean, just one type of bean that was chosen here for nutritional information, has a particularly high amount of fiber and is a good example of the healthy attributes of beans.

Tofu is bean curd. It is produced by first coagulating soy milk and then pressing the solids into squares or blocks, which are then cut up. This is similar to the way cheese is made from milk. Tofu has a mild taste and, therefore, can be used in a wide variety of sweet or savory culinary dishes. Like whole beans, tofu is low in calories and high in protein. The fat content is mostly MUFA and PUFA.

Nutritional Information for Navy Beans:	
Serving size	*½ cup (4 oz; 91 grams), cooked*
Total calories	*128*
Protein (grams)	*7.5 (high biological quality)*
Fat (grams; type)	*0.6*
Carbohydrate (grams)	*24*
Fiber (grams)	*9.6*
Other benefits	*folate 128 mcg (32%)* *thiamine 0.2 mg (15%)* *other B-complex vitamins calcium, iron, magnesium, manganese, potassium, copper, zinc, selenium, and phosphorus*

Nutritional Information for Tofu:	
Serving size	*3 oz (1" slice; 84 grams) tofu*
Total calories	*121.8*
Protein (grams)	*13.2 (high biological quality)*
Fat (grams; type)	*7.2 (MUFA 1.5 – PUFA 4.2)*
Carbohydrate (grams)	*3.6*
Fiber (grams)	*1.8*
Other benefits	*relatively high in manganese and selenium; may be prepared with calcium sulfate*

Comparisons (one ½ cup serving each)		
Cooked Bean	*calories*	*fiber (g)*
Baked beans, canned	133	7
Black	113	7.5
Black-eyed pea (cowpea)	100	5.6
Broadbeans (Fava)	93	4.6
Chickpeas (Garbanzo)	134	6.2
Lentil	115	7.8
Lima, large	108	6.6
Peas, green	67	4.4
Pinto	122	7.7
Red kidney	112	6.5
Soybean	149	5.1
White	125	5.6
Yellow	127	9.2

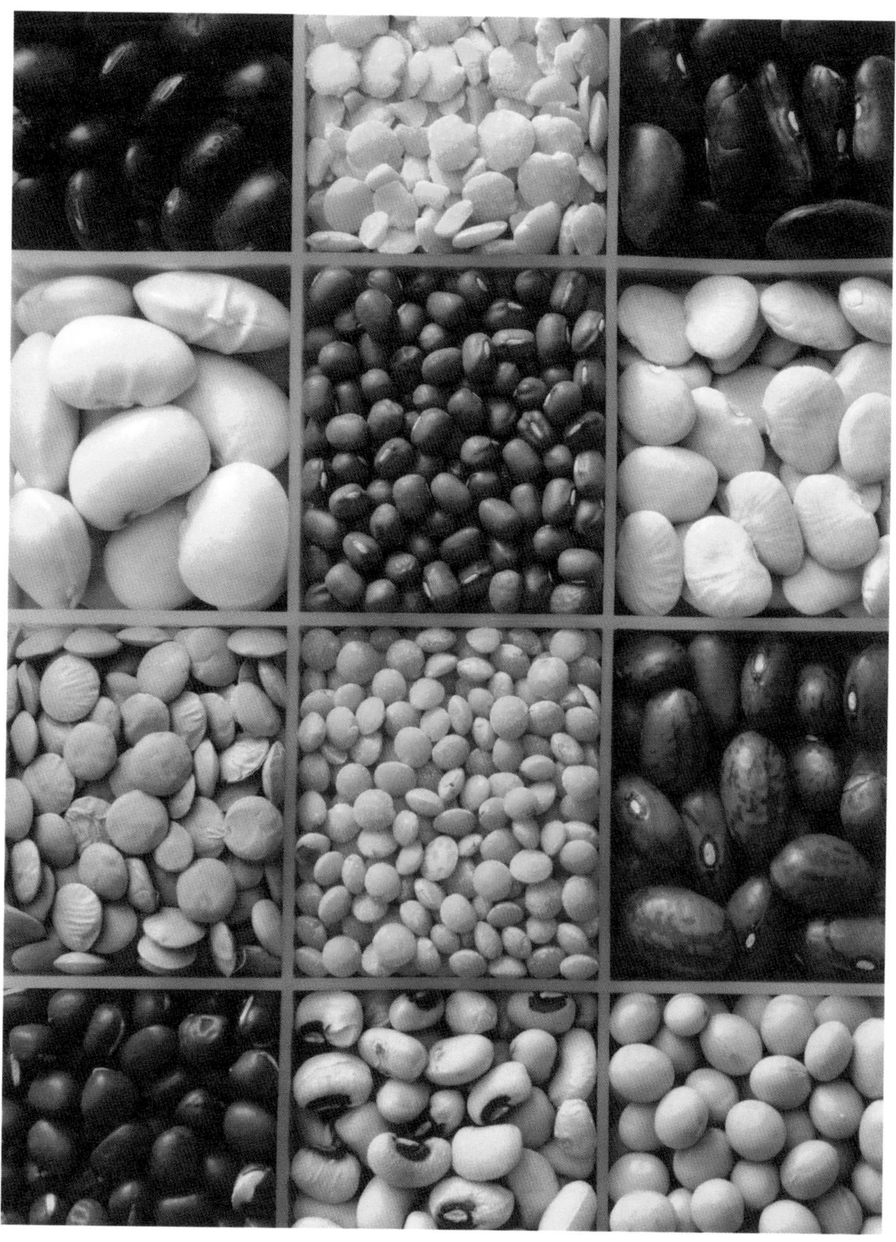

Power of Prevention Healthy Food #5: BLUEBERRIES

Blueberries are a healthy food due to the high fiber content and relatively low calories. They are also an excellent source of vitamin K, vitamin C, and the mineral manganese, and are chock full of antioxidants. These antioxidants are phyto- (plant-derived) chemicals that are associated with anti-inflammatory, anti-cancer, and lipid-lowering activities in many scientific studies. Examples of phytochemicals with antioxidant properties in blueberries are anthocyanins, proanthocyanidins, resveratrol (the same antioxidant found in red wine), flavonols, tannins, and other pigments that are responsible for the dark purple color. In general, foods that are red, orange, blue, green, yellow, and purple have phytochemicals that have antioxidant properties.

Berries are a great food to eat anytime of day. Fresh can be very satisfying as a dessert or snack between meals when trying to cut calories. When comparing the different kinds of berries, blackberries and raspberries have the greatest amounts of fiber relative to total carbohydrates. Cranberries and strawberries are also low in total carbohydrates and sugar. Fresh cherries are relatively high in total carbohydrates and sugars compared with the other berries but still make a healthy snack.

Nutritional Information for Blueberries:	
Serving size	*1 cup (148 g) raw*
Total calories	*84.4*
Protein (grams)	*1.1 gram*
Fat (grams)	*0.5*
Carbohydrate (grams)	*21.4*
Fiber (grams)	*3.6*
Other benefits	*vitamin K 28.6 mcg (36% daily needs)* *Vitamin C 14.4 mg (24% daily needs)* *Manganese 0.5 mg (25% daily needs)*

Comparisons (1 cup serving each):					
Berry	*Calories*	*Protein (g)*	*Fat (g)*	*Carbohydrate (g)*	*Fiber (g)*
Blackberry	*61.9*	*2.0*	*0.7*	*14.7*	*7.6*
Cherry	*86.9*	*1.5*	*0.3*	*22.1*	*2.9*
Cranberry	*46.0*	*0.4*	*0.1*	*12.2*	*4.6*
Raspberry	*64.0*	*1.5*	*0.8*	*14.7*	*8.0*
Strawberry	*48.6*	*1.0*	*0.5*	*11.7*	*3.0*

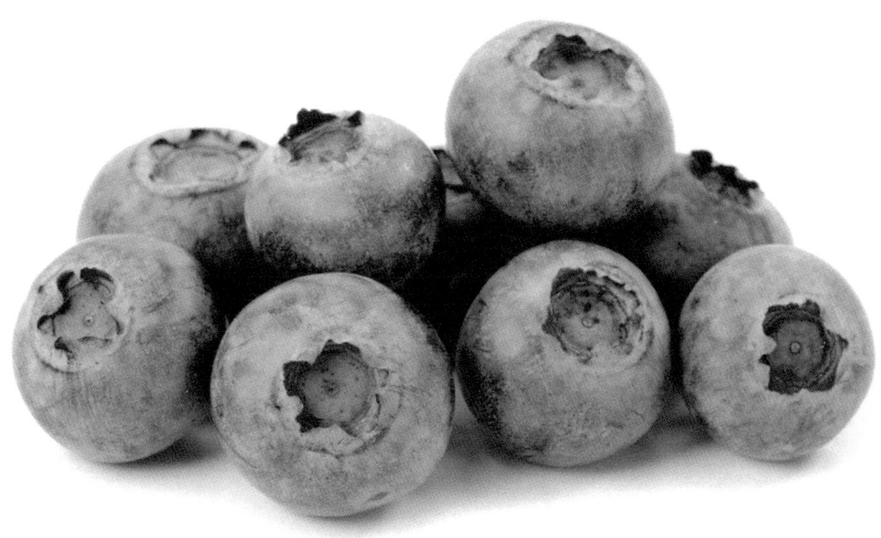

Power of Prevention Healthy Food #6: COTTAGE CHEESE, LOW-FAT

Dairy products or milk products contain a relatively high amount of high biological value protein and a relatively low amount of carbohydrate, which is primarily in the form of lactose with variable amounts of fat. These products are primarily derived from cows, but goat and sheep cheeses are also widely available. Dairy products include milk-based beverages with varying amounts of milk fat in them: whole milk, 1 to 2 percent low-fat milk, or skim (0 percent) milk, as well as higher fat-content liquids such as heavy cream. Other dairy products, including yogurt, sour cream, and cheeses, can also be high-fat, low-fat, or no-fat. Some people have a problem digesting lactose and need to limit or even avoid dairy products, or ingest lactose-digesting bacteria, which are called "probiotics" (acidophilus is a popular probiotic, but there are several others that are equally or more effective). Many lactose-free dairy products are also available.

Cottage cheese is a particularly high-protein, low-fat, low-calorie dairy product, which is an excellent addition to a healthy eating plan for most people. Cottage cheese is a cheese curd product that was developed in "cottages" from the milk product after the butter was made. The leftover curds are drained to remove liquids and leave the bulk of the "casein" protein as well as some of the "whey" protein. The curd is washed to remove the acidity and leave a mild somewhat sweet taste. Cottage cheese curds can be small with higher acid or they can be large ("chunk-style") with lower acid. When pressed, this dairy product is referred to as "farmer cheese." Cottage cheese is typically eaten alone, with fruits, or in salads. It can also be substituted for higher fat cheeses in various dishes like lasagna, stuffed shells, or even cheesecake. Farmer cheese and cottage cheese are also classically used in blintzes.

Nutritional Information for Low-Fat Cottage Cheese:	
Serving size	*4 oz (1/2 cup; 113 ounces)*
Total calories	*81.4*
Protein (grams)	*14.0 (high biological value)*
Fat (grams)	*1.2*
Carbohydrate (grams)	*3.1*
Fiber (grams)	*0*
Other benefits	*riboflavin 0.2 mg (11% daily needs)* *vit. B12 0.7 mcg (12% daily needs)* *Also high in phosphorus, sodium and selenium*
Comparisons	*whole milk cottage cheese has 116 calories, 5 g of fat, 14 g protein and nonfat cottage cheese has only 96 calories with no fat and 20 grams protein*

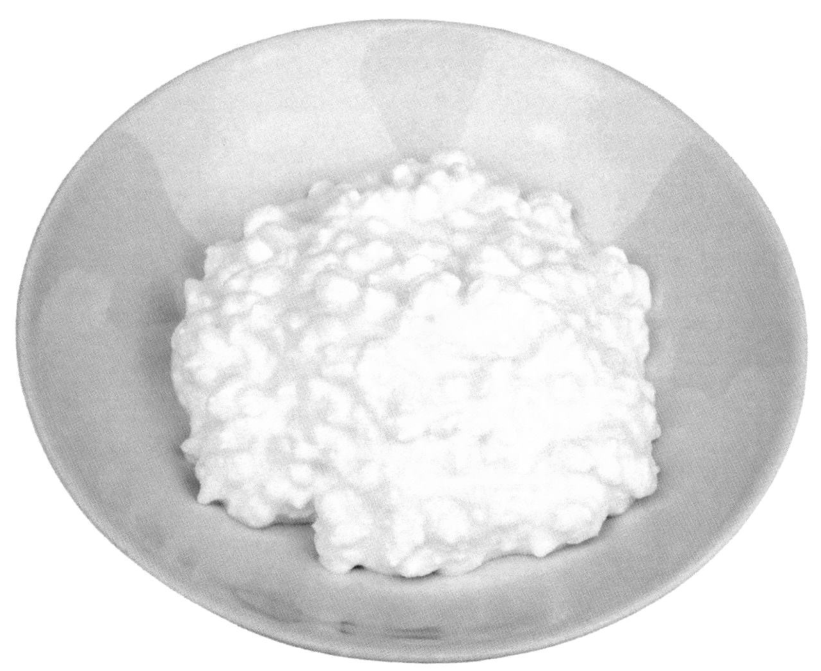

Power of Prevention Healthy Food #7: EGG

Chicken eggs are widely available and can be eaten for virtually any meal or snack. Eggs are a rich source of the highest biological value protein, ovalbumin. Egg yolk is a rich source of biotin, which is a B-complex vitamin involved in sugar and fat metabolism. Ironically, raw egg white contains a biotin-binding protein named "avidin," which, if consumed in large quantities (as raw egg whites without the biotin-rich yolk), can induce a biotin-deficiency state. This deficiency state does not occur with the consumption of cooked eggs.

There is some controversy concerning the net health risks and benefits of eating raw eggs since there is concern about salmonella-induced diarrhea. However, some people favor eating raw eggs because of the creation of proteins that cause allergies, which result from cooking the egg. In addition, some culinary recipes call for raw eggs as ingredients, such as a Hollandaise sauce, Caesar salad dressing, and the Italian dessert tiramisu. Overall, it is not necessary to eat raw eggs deliberately in order to have a healthy diet.

Egg yolks are a high source of dietary cholesterol (212 mg or 71 percent of daily needs per large [50 g] egg). Some people with high cholesterol will need to limit their intake of egg yolks. However, cooked egg whites, such as in an egg-white omelet with vegetables, can be part of a healthy, low-cholesterol diet. Another alternative is to add one whole egg to two whites for a lower cholesterol meal with little alteration in taste. Many restaurants will agree to prepare egg-white-only omelets often for a small increase in price.

Nutritional Information for Eggs:	
Serving size	*one large (50 g) egg, hard boiled*
Total calories	*77.5*
Protein (grams)	*6.3 (high biological value)*
Fat (gram; type)	*5.3; MUFA 2.0 – PUFA 0.7*
Carbohydrate (grams)	*0.6*
Fiber (grams)	*0*
Other benefits	*high in B-complex vitamins and vitamin A, selenium and phosphorus*
Comparisons	*Size/weights of eggs are: jumbo (>71g), extra large (64-71g), large (57-63g), medium (50-56g), small (43-49g), and peewee (35-42g)*

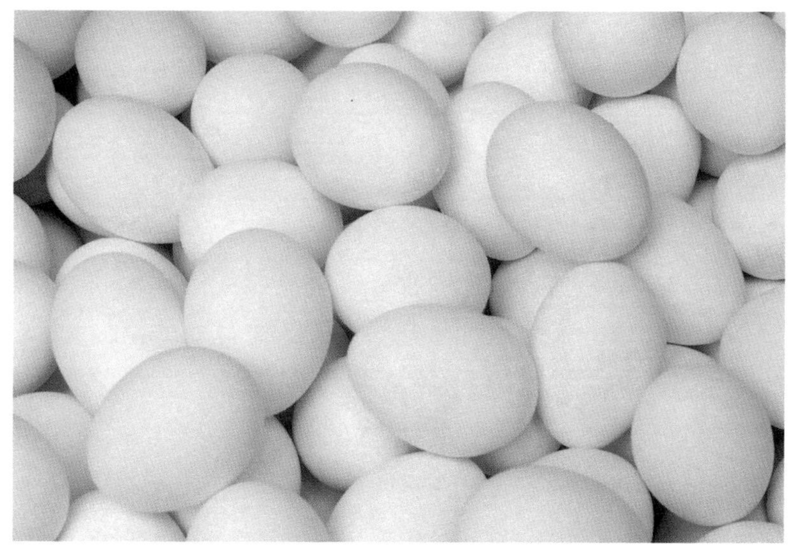

Power of Prevention Healthy Food #8: OLIVES

The health benefits of whole olives are mainly related to their relatively low calorie composition and high MUFA and PUFA content. Olives are the fruit of an evergreen tree or shrub and represent a principal agricultural product of eastern Mediterranean, Asian, and African regions. Olives are their natural green color when harvested and then ripen to a dark purple color. Freshly picked olives contain certain nonpoisonous chemicals, called "phenolic compounds," which make the fruit have a bad taste and unsuitable for eating. All olives undergo fermentation in brine solution, which preserves them and increases their palatability.

A serving size for ripe olives is 15 grams with approximately 25 calories per serving; this corresponds to six small, five medium, four large, three extra large or jumbo, two colossal, or one super colossal olive. Olive oil is also a very healthy choice as salad dressing or in food preparation. Olive oil is also part of the Mediterranean diet. Approximately two tablespoons (23 grams) of olive oil per day can provide the various heart and blood vessel health benefits of the Mediterranean diet.

Nutritional Information for Olives:	
Serving size	*15 g (3 extra large black olives)*
Total calories	*21*
Protein (grams)	*0.2*
Fat (grams; type)	*2 (MUFA 1.5 g – PUFA 0.2 g)*
Carbohydrate (grams)	*1*
Fiber (grams)	*0.6*

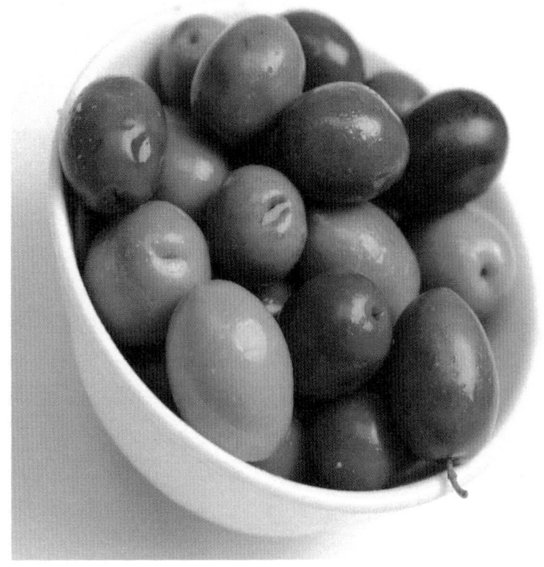

Power of Prevention Healthy Food #9: QUINOA

Quinoa (pronounced KEEN-wah) is the seed of the goosefoot plant indigenous to South America. It is an ancient food that has been consumed for thousands of years but has only recently become popular in this country. Quinoa is considered to be 100 percent whole grain although it is not truly a grain, but rather a seed. Quinoa is particularly high in protein (12–18 percent) and is a complete protein as it contains eight essential amino acids. It is also high in fiber, containing 7 grams per 100 grams, and is high in B vitamins, vitamin E, iron, magnesium, and phosphorus.

Quinoa is sold dry in a box. It is pre-rinsed to remove certain bitter chemicals called "saponins." The dry quinoa is cooked like rice, simmered in water or in a rice cooker. The cooked product is light and fluffy with a slightly nutty taste. Quinoa is oft1en prepared with herbs or spices and served warm as a carbohydrate side dish with a dinner meal as an alternative to rice or couscous. It can also be served cold in salads or added to soups. Sometimes it is sweetened with honey and berries and served for breakfast. Quinoa is an excellent addition to a vegetarian diet as a protein source and is gluten-free and, therefore, safe for people with celiac disease. Quinoa seeds can be ground into flour, which can then be used for pasta, pancakes, or baked goods.

Nutritional Information for Quinoa:	
Serving size	*50 grams*
Total calories	*188*
Protein (grams)	*7*
Fat (grams; type)	*3 (saturated fat 1 g)*
Carbohydrate (grams)	*35*
Fiber (grams)	*3*
Other benefits	*B-vitamins, vitamin E, iron*

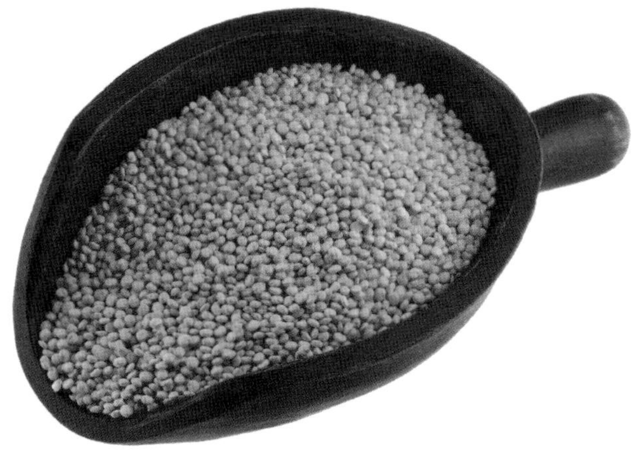

Power of Prevention Healthy Food #10: SALMON

Fresh fish, especially oily cold-water fish, offers unique health advantages while providing a protein component to a healthy meal. Fish is high in protein, low in saturated fat, and high in MUFA, PUFA, and omega-3 fatty acids (n-3 FA), which are associated with anti-inflammatory and lipid-lowering benefits.

Among the extensive varieties of fish readily available as food in the US, salmon is among the most popular. Salmon are found in the Atlantic and Pacific oceans as well as the Great Lakes and other smaller landlocked lakes. Farmed salmon may have lower amounts of n-3 FA and higher amounts of environmental toxins called dioxins (polychlorinated biphenyls [PCBs] are an example of dioxins). However, scientific studies have shown that the benefits of eating farmed salmon still outweigh any dangers from these contaminants. In general, Atlantic salmon are mostly farmed and Pacific salmon are mostly wild. Another difference between wild and farmed salmon is the natural color of the meat. Wild salmon meat is naturally orange to red, owing to the natural vitamin A-related chemicals, called carotenoids, in the small shellfish the salmon eats. On the other hand, farmed salmon have naturally white meat due to the food they are given, but frequently these farms will add certain chemicals that can make the farmed salmon meat pinkish. Besides fresh and frozen, salmon is also available as a canned product and as "lox" or "gravlax," which has been cured in salt and sometimes sugar and spices and then sometimes cold-smoked.

There has been much attention paid to the mercury content of salmon and other fish. This is especially important to many health-conscious people who have deliberately increased their fish consumption in order to avoid meats with saturated fats. The mercury contamination of various edible fish is provided in the table below. As can be seen, tilefish from the Gulf of Mexico, king mackerel, orange roughy, shark, and swordfish are particularly high in mercury content. In non-pregnant adults, the potential for mercury intoxication and physical harm should not outweigh the benefits from a healthy diet that incorporates fish.

Fish	*Mercury (parts per million)*
Anchovies	*0.04*
Grouper	*0.46*
Haddock	*0.03*
Halibut	*0.25*
Herring	*0.04*
Mackerel, Atlantic	*0.05*
Mackerel, King	*0.73*
Mackerel, Pacific	*0.09*
Mackerel, Spanish	*0.18*
Orange Roughy	*0.55*
Salmon, canned	*not detected*
Salmon, fresh/frozen	*0.01*
Sardine	*0.02*
Shark	*0.99*

Snapper	*0.19*
Swordfish	*0.98*
Tilefish	*1.45*
Trout	*0.07*
Tuna, albacore, canned	*0.35*
Tuna, albacore, fresh/frozen	*0.36*
Whitefish	*0.07*

Source of data: FDA 1990–2004, "National Marine Fisheries Service Survey of Trace Elements in the Fishery Resource" report 1978, and "The Occurrence of Mercury in the Fishery Resources of the Gulf of Mexico" report 2000.
http://www.epa.gov/waterscience/fish/files/MethylmercuryBrochure.pdf (accessed July 17, 2008).

Nutritional Information for Salmon:	
Serving size	*½ filet (154 grams) of wild Atlantic*
	Salmon cooked with dry heat
Total calories	*280*
Protein (grams)	*39.2*
Fat (grams; type)	*12.5 (MUFA 4.2 – PUFA 5.0) with 3982 mg n-3 FA*
Carbohydrate (grams)	*0*
Fiber (grams)	*0*
Other benefits	*very high in B-complex vitamins especially niacin (15.5 mg 78% daily needs) and vitamin B12 (4.7 mcg; 78% daily needs) also high in iron, magnesium, phosphorus, potassium, zinc, copper and > 100% of daily needs for selenium (103%)*

Comparisons (comparable weight, wild unless otherwise stated, cooked with dry heat unless indicated as canned)					
Fish	*calories*	*protein-g*	*MUFA-g*	*PUFA-g*	*n-3 FA-mg*
Halibut	223	42.4	1.5	1.5	1064
Herring	290	32.9	6.8	3.9	3171
Mackerel	231	21.0	6.2	3.8	1251
Salmon, Atlantic, farmed	367	39.3	7.9	7.9	4023
Salmon, pink, canned 6 oz	236	33.6	3.0	3.4	2986
Salmon, Altantic, wild, raw	281	39.3	4.2	5.0	3996
Salmon, sockeye	335	42.3	8.2	3.7	2207
Sardine, canned 1 cup	310	36.7	5.8	7.7	2205
Swordfish	164	26.9	2.1	1.3	1120

Trout, rainbow	215	32.8	2.5	2.6	1680
Tuna, bluefin	312	50.8	3.4	3.2	2828
Tuna, white, canned in water	220	40.6	2.6	3.8	1636

Suggested reading

Nutrition Data. www.nutritiondata.com (accessed on July 17, 2008)

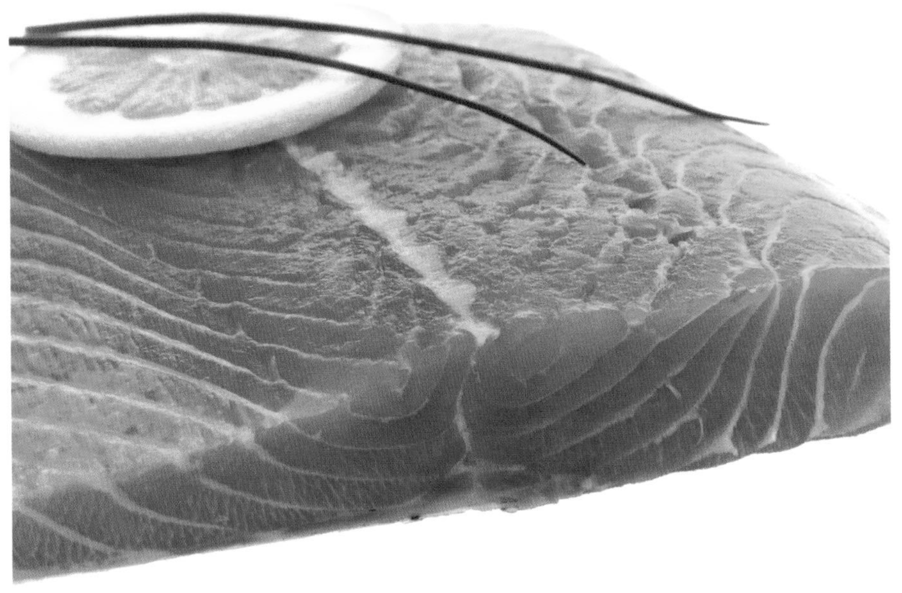

CHAPTER 2.7

Nutrition and the Culinary Arts

Elise M. Brett, MD, FACE, CNSP

Food should be an enjoyable part of life, even for those with medical problems or those who are trying to lose weight. Meal preparation and eating consumes a large part of our days. A recent survey showed that Americans spend, on average, just over an hour per day eating and drinking and additional time grocery shopping and preparing food. Furthermore, food is often at the center of formal and informal social events. Food that is prepared at home is often fresher and more nutritious than processed foods or meals consumed in restaurants. These days, Americans have easy access to a wide variety of ingredients from around the world and can easily experiment with different cuisines to keep home-cooking interesting.

A "healthy meal" is typically one that is low in saturated fat and well balanced. Most meals should contain elements of protein, fat, and carbohydrate. Fruit and vegetable portions should generally be the largest to add bulk and fiber without adding excess calories. An easy way to ensure a well-balanced meal is to make the plate contain different colors. The compounds that give fruits and vegetables their red, orange, yellow, purple, or green colors are typically the ones that provide special health benefits, so making a plate colorful is an easy way of ensuring that some of these micronutrients are included. Chefs use this method to make a meal pleasing to the eye, and even young children can understand this concept. Chefs also avoid repeating food types and textures within a meal, and they try to pair rich foods with lighter ones for balance and health.

Certain precautions need to be taken for safety when preparing foods at home. Purchased meats and fish should generally be used within forty-eight hours or frozen for future use. Fresh fish should not have a "fishy" odor, and the texture should be firm. Frozen meats should be defrosted in the refrigerator or the microwave, not at room temperature, in order to avoid the growth of bacteria. Poultry must be cooked to an internal temperature of 170°F and pork to 155°F to kill bacteria. Fruits and vegetables should not have major blemishes. They should be stored in the refrigerator to be kept freshest and should be thoroughly washed before use. Canned food should not be used if the can is dented, as this may be a sign of bacterial growth. Leftovers should be refrigerated within two hours and eaten within two to four days. One must wash his or her hands prior to and after food preparation. Cutting boards and knives, particularly those that have been in contact with uncooked poultry or eggs, should be thoroughly washed with soap. Surfaces used to cut uncooked meat should not then be used to prepare other foods until thoroughly washed with soap and hot water. Sponges used to clean pots and pans should be replaced weekly or washed in the dishwasher. Dishrags should be washed regularly as these too may accumulate bacteria.

The method of food preparation can influence the nutritional content of the meal. Grilling over direct heat or broiling under direct heat are particularly healthful methods as they usually require no additional fat or only small amounts, as in marinades. Grilling is a wonderful option for steaks, fish, chicken, and vegetables. Excess fat should be trimmed prior to cooking for health and to avoid flare-ups. When grilling beef, it is best to choose a lean cut, such as sirloin, which contains only about 150 calories in a 3-ounce portion, and keep portion sizes small.

The method of sautéing involves searing food over direct heat in a small amount of butter or oil. This is a better alternative to frying, which requires immersion in oil. Usually only one tablespoon of fat per serving is needed to sauté. For optimal results, one should avoid crowding in the pan so the food cooks evenly but also avoid using too large a pan so that the sauce does not burn. Veal or chicken cutlets or fish filets are more healthily prepared by sautéing than pan-frying or deep-frying. For an easy main course, fish, chicken, or veal cutlets can be dredged in flour and then sautéed in a little butter or oil. The sauce can be finished with lemon juice and parsley or other herbs (or capers) with or without stock or wine for a "meuniere" or "piccata-type" preparation.

Stir-frying is similar to sautéing. It is usually done with a little oil, lemon juice, chilies, and soy sauce in a wok for Asian-style recipes. Stir-fry dishes containing meats or tofu and lots of vegetables can be very satisfying and complete, low-calorie meals.

Poaching, immersion in liquid and simmering, is particularly healthful, as it requires no additional fat. Fish, chicken, eggs, or fruit can be cooked by poaching in water or a combination of water, wine, and herbs.

Roasting is cooking with indirect heat as in the oven. Roasted meats are generally "sealed" with fat to prevent drying. The skins of roasted poultry should be removed prior to eating to avoid eating excess fat. In the wintertime, roasted root vegetables prepared with a little oil with or without a bit of maple syrup are a nice accompaniment to a protein for a complete meal. Sliced potatoes can be roasted with a little oil and salt as a more healthful alterative to french fries.

Braising is an excellent, healthful choice for more tender meats such as chicken, pork, or veal and is also ideal for firm vegetables, such as artichokes, leeks, or brussels sprouts. In braising, the food is partially immersed in liquid such as water or stock with added wine, lemon juice, or vinegar to help tenderize it and cooked over direct heat. Brown braising, used for red meats, requires searing in a pan prior to braising.

One key to maximal enjoyment of healthy meals is to choose seasonal ingredients. Although most fruits and vegetables are now available anytime of the year, if not purchased in season, they are often not worth eating. The best example is the tomato, which in peak season is juicy with a slight acidic character and needs almost no accompaniment, whereas tomatoes in the winter are typically flavorless and mealy in texture. Fresh blueberries, raspberries, blackberries, and cherries in the summertime are incredibly flavorful and make a naturally sweet dessert or snack without the need to add fat or sugar. Fresh corn in the summer is one of nature's sweetest creations and can be boiled, roasted, or grilled without added fat.

Sweet peaches and plums are at their peak in the late summer and early fall. Fall squashes are easily prepared and delicious when roasted and eaten in cubes or pureed. Few foods taste better than a slightly tart, perfectly crisp, freshly picked apple that in no way resembles the supermarket varieties. Fall apples can be stored for several months in the refrigerator and will maintain their crispness.

Pomegranates are a special fall/winter treat that are low in calories and high in vitamins and antioxidants. Citrus fruits, such as grapefruits and oranges, can be shipped from Florida groves all winter and early spring when most other fruits are not at their peak.

In spring, it is fun to experiment with new preparations of artichokes, asparagus, and fava beans for interesting side dishes. Strawberries are one of the earliest spring fruits. Fresh from the farm stand, strawberries are markedly different and better tasting than the firm supermarket varieties. Berries purchased off-season typically cost two to three times their seasonal price. Fresh berries can be frozen in the summer for use in low-fat desserts or fruit smoothies all year round.

Americans often have green salads as a starter as opposed to the Europeans who have them after the meal. Starting a meal with a green salad adds bulk, fiber, and vitamins without adding excess calories. Salads should be dressed with homemade vinaigrettes or reduced-calorie store-bought versions. Thick, mayonnaise-based salad dressings such as Thousand Island or blue cheese, popular only in America and Britain, should generally be avoided. These dressings add loads of calories and "cover up" rather than enhance the flavor of the vegetables. A simple vinaigrette can be prepared using one part olive oil to three or four parts vinegar. Vinegar, salt, pepper, and a spoonful of Dijon mustard are whisked in a bowl, and the oil is slowly drizzled in while whisking to emulsify. Fresh herbs, shallots, or other dried spices can be added for more variety, and different flavor vinegars can be tried. Vinegar has actually been shown to decrease hunger and may help one to consume less food later in the meal.

Hot soups or chilis are wonderful starters or main courses for fall or winter meals. It is best to choose soups that do not contain heavy cream in their base. Pureed vegetable soups such as butternut squash, pea, lentil, or mushroom are filling and do not require cream to thicken them. Spicy chilis can be made with a variety of vegetables and beans for a lower calorie, higher fiber, yet equally flavorful version of the traditional meat chili. In summertime, fresh cold gazpacho is easily prepared by pureeing fresh tomatoes, cucumbers, and bell peppers in the food processor and then seasoning with vinegar, lime or lemon, and Tabasco sauce or jalapenos. The dish is easy to prepare, tasty, and nutritious with a minimal amount of calories.

Sauces for meats, fish, vegetables, and pasta can add flavor and elegance to a meal, but are often the major source of calories and saturated fat. It is best to avoid sauces that are based with heavy cream or those made with a full stick or two of butter. Alternatively, a French velouté-type sauce made with chicken stock and flour, just a tablespoon of butter, and fresh herbs is an elegant and healthy choice. Plain-yogurt-based, Indian-spiced sauces are a particularly healthful and unique choice. Pureed roasted red peppers make a colorful, healthy sauce for fish or pasta. Chopped vegetable salsas are also flavorful over fish or chicken without adding significant calories. Tomato sauces are generally a good option. Tasty homemade sauces can be made any time of the year using canned Italian (San Marzano) plum tomatoes, olive oil, onions, basil, and salt. For meat sauces, one can choose a lean sirloin over a chuck or consider substituting ground turkey for ground beef to reduce fat content without sacrificing flavor.

Salt is essential in cooking and should not be eliminated from recipes, as it brings out the flavor of most foods. The relationship between dietary salt and hypertension remains unclear and controversial. Although a subset of people with hypertension may be particularly "salt-sensitive," it is probably not necessary to restrict salt in the general population or in all patients with treated hypertension. However, salty snacks such as chips should be limited since they contain high amounts of salt and lots of calories with little nutritional value. Other processed foods, such as frozen dinners, soups, or cured meats, are best limited as these generally are very high in sodium and low in nutritional value. Fresh or frozen vegetables are preferable to canned vegetables as the latter contain very high amounts of unnecessary sodium. Many chefs recommend cooking with a salt with coarser crystals such as kosher salt or sea salt as it is easier to pinch and sprinkle just the right amount. One should never need to add salt to a dish at the table. Spices should be used generously when cooking as they add flavor, limit the need for salt, and do not affect the nutritional content of a meal.

In summary, the wide availability of fresh produce and imported products makes cooking at home exciting and well suited for the health conscious. Lots of superb free recipes are available on the Internet (see Suggested Readings below). In general, it is best to spend a little more for quality ingredients and keep portion sizes down. Purchasing seasonal ingredients usually guarantees the best flavor and also the lowest cost.

Suggested Readings

Center for Nutrition Policy and Promotion, US Department of Agriculture. "Dietary Guidelines for Americans 2005." www.healthierus.gov/dietaryguidelines (accessed on October 18, 2008).

Epicurious. www.epicurious.com (accessed August 23, 2008).

Food Network. www.foodnetwork.com (accessed August 23, 2008).

Chapter 3.1

Nutrition for the Newborn and Infant

Jason M. Hollander, M.D., C.N.S.P.

Nutrition in the First Year of Life

Adequate nutrition in the first year of life is necessary to ensure normal growth and development and to avoid illness. Unlike older children and adults whose diets are usually constant, the diet of an infant changes dramatically over the first twelve months. This reflects changes in the nervous system, dental development, and the specific nutritional needs of infancy. A newborn will drink about 3 ounces of breast milk or formula every two to three hours throughout the day and night. By four to six months, an infant will have developed the head control and oral motor skills to begin eating solid food. By one year, an infant will eat most table foods.

Throughout the first year of life, caloric intake must meet basic energy needs as well as provide enough energy to support the dramatic growth of infancy. A normal one-month-old grows about 1 centimeter per week and gains about 30 grams (1 ounce) per day. An average newborn weighs 3.5 kilograms (7.7 pounds). Most infants will double their birth weight by four months and triple their birth weight by one year of age. Early in the postnatal period, organs increase in size as their cells divide. Failure to meet the energy requirements of increased cell division may impair growth and lead to permanent damage to the brain, nerves, and other organ systems.

Infants communicate their needs to their caregivers and will rarely settle down when hungry. Thus, it is rare that a healthy newborn will be underfed. The weight and height of infants are followed closely, as are important developmental milestones. When these parameters deviate from expected norms, an evaluation is typically instituted by a pediatrician. Commonly, adverse social circumstances are responsible for abnormal growth and development. Rarely, a medical illness can be identified. For the vast majority of infants, proper feeding and nutrition can be easily implemented as long as common sense and basic guidelines are observed (see table 1).

Formulas

The American Academy of Pediatrics recommends that breast-feeding be the preferred feeding for all infants. However, in the absence of human milk, iron-fortified formulas are a reasonable substitute for feeding the healthy full-term infant throughout the first year of life. Despite the many advances in formulas over the last seventy years, today's formulas still do not duplicate the composition of human milk, which also contains hormones, immunologic agents, enzymes, and live cells.

Most infants thrive on standard cow milk-based formulas, but real differences do exist between human milk and modern formulas. The protein *quality* and *content* of human milk differs substantially from that of cow milk. Human milk contains less protein but more of the easily digested whey protein than cow milk. Additionally, the amino acid profile in human milk is markedly different than that of other animals (see chapter 2.3 on Protein). For instance, taurine is an amino acid that is important to nerve and brain growth in humans. Cow milk is completely deficient in taurine; therefore, taurine must be added to infant formulas in order to ensure normal growth.

Fat makes up about 50 percent of breast milk as well as cow milk-based formulas. Most manufacturers of infant formulas replace some or all of the butterfat of cow milk with a mixture of vegetable oils to improve fat digestibility and absorption. The optimal composition of fat in commercial formulas remains an area of great interest, particularly with regard to major types of fatty acids: omega-3 and omega-6 fatty acids. For example, manufacturers commonly add the omega-3 fatty acid "doxosahexaenoic acid" (abbreviated as DHA) and the omega-6 fatty acid "arachidonic acid" (abbreviated as ARA) to infant formulas. Both DHA and ARA are not present in appreciable quantities in cow milk but are present in human milk. Some evidence suggests that these fatty acids are important for the developing nervous system and vision.

Human milk and cow milk-based formulas are also different in terms of the iron content. A normal infant needs about 1,500 milligrams of iron in the first year of life. This is equivalent to 8 to 10 milligrams per day. Most formulas supply 10 to 12 milligrams per day, but human milk only has a fraction of this amount. Surprisingly, infants that are only breast-fed are not iron deficient. This is because there is better iron absorption from breast milk than there is from cows' milk. Low-iron formulas are also available, but there is no role for these formulas in infant feeding. It is widely believed that the iron in infant formulas causes constipation, but there is no evidence to support this. In fact, the use of these low-iron formulas can actually lead to anemia. Other nutrients like zinc, selenium, chromium, calcium, phosphorous, and various vitamins are present in adequate amounts in infant formulas even though their optimal intake amounts are unknown.

Soy-Based Formulas

Soy-based formulas have been available since the 1960s and support infant growth similar to both human milk and cow milk-based formulas. The ratio of fat, carbohydrate, and protein in soy-based formulas is the same as in milk-based formulas. Of course, the protein source is soy, rather than casein and whey, and the carbohydrate source is sucrose or cornstarch hydrolysates, rather than lactose. The fats in soy formulas, however, are quite similar to cow milk-based formulas.

Soy formulas may be used by strict vegetarians. At times, infants who are allergic to milk proteins are switched to soy. This maneuver is somewhat controversial. Between 20 and 80 percent of infants who are allergic to casein are also allergic to soy. Soy formulas are ideal for infants who are unable to process the carbohydrate in milk (as with the disorders "lactase deficiency" and "galactosemia") and may in certain situations improve diarrhea following a stomach or intestine infection. Finally, many infants are tried on soy formulas when they are experiencing "colic" (pain), spitting up, or vomiting. Most of the time, these problems are unrelated to the formula; however, a small number of infants will respond for unclear reasons.

Protein Hydrolysate Formulas

Protein hydrolysate formulas were designed for infants with severe milk and soy protein allergies or who cannot effectively digest standard formulas due to certain illnesses. The protein in these formulas is extensively digested (or "hydrolyzed") into amino acids and small proteins called peptides, which are less likely to cause an allergic reaction in certain children.

Most hydrolysate formulas are lactose free. Manufacturers use sucrose, tapioca starch, corn syrup, and cornstarch in various mixtures. Fat in these formulas is comprised of primarily medium chain fatty acids to optimize absorption. In general, protein hydrolysate formulas are recommended as the preferred feeding for infants intolerant of cow milk or soy protein or for those with significant absorption problems.

Breast-feeding

Human milk is designed specifically for the growth of human infants. The macronutrient (protein, carbohydrate, and fat) content of human milk has been discussed above. This section will focus on the other components of human milk as well as the psychological and health benefits of breast-feeding.

Living cells are present in high concentrations in human milk. Cells called macrophages and lymphocytes help to fight infection and boost the immunity of the newborn. Immunoglobulins are specialized proteins designed to latch onto bacteria and kill them. These proteins are an important part of breast milk and provide immunological protection in the infant's intestines.

Other factors found in breast milk include nucleotides, which boost immunity and enhance gastrointestinal health; lactoferrin, which possesses antimicrobial properties; and enzymes (proteins that accelerate chemical reactions), which can neutralize invading bacteria.

A number of growth factors, including the "epidermal growth factor," "transforming growth factor," and "nerve growth factor" are also present in human milk. As their names imply, these factors are important for the growth and development of certain types of cells. Countless other substances are present in human milk including "resistance factor," "interferon," and "complement"; the exact role of these substances in human milk is not understood.

The Benefits of Breast-feeding

A large body of evidence exists demonstrating the health benefits of breast-feeding. Breast-fed infants are much less likely to develop common infections. Breast-fed infants may have as few as half the number of ear infections as formula-fed infants. Gastrointestinal infections and deep respiratory infections are also less common and/or less severe among breast-fed infants. Some evidence even suggests that breast-feeding for four to six months may provide relative protection against certain diseases such as celiac sprue, type 1 diabetes, inflammatory conditions of the intestine, certain cancers, allergic conditions, and obesity.

Breast-feeding also enhances mother-infant bonding. Interestingly, some evidence suggests that breast-feeding mothers tend to demonstrate less anxiety, depression, fatigue, and guilt than mothers who choose to formula feed. Moreover, mothers who breast-feed often report greater satisfaction surrounding the feeding experience. Overall, breast-feeding is emotionally and physiologically the optimal feeding for most neonates and infants.

Food Allergies

Adverse food reactions can be divided into true allergic reactions and all other reactions (see chapter 4.14, "Food Allergies"). Twenty to 30 percent of individuals will report a food allergy in themselves or their children. However, a true food allergy is present in only 6 to 8 percent of children less than five years of age. A food allergy is an immunologic response toward food proteins. Some reactions are acute and potentially life-threatening, while others occur chronically and are frequently isolated to the gastrointestinal tract.

Symptoms of an acute reaction include hives, swelling of the lips and eyes, wheezing, nausea, abdominal pain, vomiting, diarrhea, difficulty breathing, low blood pressure, and even death. Chronic allergic conditions can present with failure to grow appropriately. Additionally, blood may be found in the stool. Fortunately, signs and symptoms of chronic allergic reactions can rapidly improve when the inciting food protein is avoided.

Asthma and atopic dermatitis (eczema) are related conditions in which food may play a role in some babies and children. When asthma and/or eczema are not well controlled with reasonable standard therapy, consultation with a pediatric allergist is recommended.

Common dietary allergens include peanuts, tree nuts, milk, eggs, wheat, soy, and shellfish. Fortunately, most children outgrow common and hard-to-avoid allergens like milk and eggs. Certain other allergies tend to persist, like those to nuts and seafood.

Regardless of the allergy, it is important that allergies be viewed as a serious medical condition that can be life-threatening, even if past reactions have seemed "mild." Preparation and education are important. All caregivers of allergic infants and children must be trained to use an emergency epinephrine injection. In addition, every effort must be made to prevent the accidental ingestion of a known allergen. However, if such ingestion occurs, the outcome will be favorable as long as timely medical care is provided.

How Can You Tell If Your Baby Has a Nutritional Problem?

During the first year of life, infants are examined frequently to ensure normal growth and development and to address concerns that parents may have. Most pediatricians will see a newborn within one week to one month after delivery. Following this visit, an infant will be seen again at two months, four months, six months, nine months, and one year. At each visit, length, weight, and head circumference will be plotted on graphs to ensure that growth is as predicted. At each visit, the pediatrician will also ask developmental questions and may perform simple tests to confirm that development is also progressing normally. If growth parameters begin to progress too slowly, or not at all, then a condition known as "failure to thrive" is recognized and the pediatrician will evaluate the infant for common conditions that can impair growth. Fortunately, the majority of cases are amenable to nutritional and/or pharmacologic intervention, and growth can eventually be restored to normal.

Table 1. Suggested feeding schedule for infants

Age	Food
0-6 months	Breast milk or formula only
6-7 months	Iron fortified cereal (rice, oatmeal) – in a bowl w/ a spoon
	Mashed fruit
7-8 months	Mashed vegetables
8-9 months	Finger foods (Cheerios, well cooked carrots, bananas)
9 months	Pureed meats, poultry
10 months	Cooked table foods, cut into small pieces
12 months	All table foods

1. New foods should not be introduced more frequently than every 3-5 days to ensure no allergy exists.
2. Peanuts, hard candies, grapes, popcorn and other such foods must not be given to infants as they pose a serious choking hazard.
3. Children at high risk for developing food allergies may benefit from avoiding highly allergenic foods until after the age of 2 years; consultation with an allergist is recommended if your child is at high risk for food allergies.

Suggested Readings

BBC.home. "Nutrition: Life stages." http://www.bbc.co.uk/health/healthy_living/nutrition/life_infant1.shtml (accessed on September 30, 2008).

CNN.com. "Feeding your newborn: Remember the basics." http://www.cnn.com/HEALTH/library/PR/00057.html (accessed on September 30, 2008).

Faqs.org. "Infant nutrition." http://www.faqs.org/nutrition/Hea-Irr/Infant-Nutrition.html (accessed on September 30, 2008).

Medline Plus. "Infant and newborn care." http://www.nlm.nih.gov/medlineplus/infantandnewborncare.html (accessed on September 30, 2008).

United States Department of Agriculture. "Life cycle nutrition: Infant nutrition." http://fnic.nal.usda.gov/nal_display/index.php?info_center=4&tax_level=2&tax_subject=257&topic_id=1352 (accessed on September 30, 2008).

Chapter 3.2

Nutrition for Children and Adolescents

Jason M. Hollander, MD, CNSP

The Basics

Food is plentiful in this country, so much so that children are unknowingly being overfed high-calorie, sweetened, prepackaged, artificial foods. At the same time, physical education programs are being cut and more time is spent in cyberspace than on soccer fields and tennis courts. Mindless eating in front of computer screens and television sets accounts for hundreds of empty calories consumed every day by American children. Obesity is a public health crisis, and sadly, it has not spared the young people in this country. Nearly one in five young people aged two to nineteen are overweight, and this number is on the rise. Hardest hit are certain ethnic minorities including African Americans, Hispanic Americans, and American Indians. The easiest way to reverse this alarming trend is to teach the littlest members of our society how to eat right and stay active.

What Is a Balanced Diet?

A healthy and balanced diet for children and adolescents emphasizes fruits and vegetables, whole grains, lean meats and fish, legumes (peas, nuts, and beans), and low-fat dairy products. Typical American staples like pizza or hamburgers tend to be calorie dense, high in salt, loaded with unhealthy saturated and *trans* fat, and essentially without fiber. Diets higher in vegetables, fruits, and whole grains tend to be very low in salt, high in potassium, high in magnesium, and high in fiber. These healthy diets reduce the risk of obesity, hypertension, heart disease, and certain types of cancer.

Dairy

Low-fat dairy products are an important part of a balanced diet. Dairy products are high in calcium. Adequate calcium intake is necessary to optimize the integrity of growing bones. In general, after the age of two years, there is no role for full-fat dairy products in the diet. It is recommended that all milk consumed after this age be fat-free or skim milk. Similarly, low-fat cheeses, yogurt, and cottage cheese are excellent sources of protein and calcium. Moreover, some evidence suggests that low-fat dairy products prevent overweight and obesity.

Meat and Beans

Lean meats and fish that are baked, broiled, grilled, or steamed provide complete protein to support growth. The consumption of adequate protein calories is particularly important during periods of rapid growth like adolescence. Additionally, protein provides a more durable satiety when compared to high-carbohydrate foods.

Other important sources of protein include nuts, seeds, peas, and beans. Some nuts and seeds are high in essential fatty acids and antioxidants like vitamin E. Dry beans and peas are excellent sources of protein as well. However, they are also high in important nutrients like zinc, iron, and soluble fiber. Many people choose only red meat and chicken to supply their dietary protein. Varying food choices will boost the intake of essential fats and other nutrients. Including fish, turkey, a variety of different beans, and various nuts in the diet does this.

Whole Grains

There has been much focus during the last several years directed at the health benefits of whole-grain products as compared to their refined counterparts. Whole grains are cereal grains that are not processed. Therefore, they retain the bran and germ that are naturally high in minerals (magnesium, manganese, phosphorous, and selenium), vitamins (B6, niacin, and vitamin E), protein, and fiber. Refined grains are stripped of the bran and germ components and do not have these nutrients.

Unfortunately, the food industry has confused consumers to some degree with misleading labeling. "Contains whole wheat," "100% wheat," and "multigrain" are phrases that may appear on food labels and in no way guarantee that a food is made primarily from whole grain. The label must read "whole wheat bread" or "whole wheat pasta" to ensure that you are purchasing a whole-grain product.

Dietary fiber from whole grains helps to reduce cholesterol and the risk of heart disease. Fiber also improves intestinal health, reduces the risk of an intestinal disease called "diverticulosis," and possibly protects against colon cancer. Finally, high-fiber foods such as whole grains provide a feeling of fullness with fewer calories. This can help prevent overeating, which is important to maintaining a healthy weight.

Fruits and Vegetables

Fruits and vegetables are underconsumed in this country. Americans frequently choose to snack on prepackaged items like cookies and crackers. Fruits and vegetables provide a number of important nutrients, and people who eat more of these foods are less likely to develop certain diseases. A diet high in fruits and vegetables reduces the risk of developing high blood pressure, type 2 diabetes, obesity, and stroke. Additionally, a diet high in fruits and vegetables may protect against gastrointestinal cancers. Fruits and vegetables are important sources of potassium, fiber, vitamin C, vitamin A, vitamin E, and folate. The amount of fruits and vegetables one needs depends on age, gender, and physical activity; however, a good rule of thumb is to have one or even two fresh fruits or vegetables with every meal and more during the day as snacks.

Fats

While fat does not constitute a food group, "healthy fat" is an important part of a balanced diet. In general, unhealthy fats, like saturated fats (found mostly in animal products) and *trans* fats (found in many baked goods), should be limited as they elevate unhealthy cholesterol in the blood and increase the risk for heart disease. Healthy fats, on the other hand, can be found in fish, nuts, and certain oils, like canola oil and olive oil. Healthy fats may promote longevity. However, all fats are relatively high in calories, so even healthy fats can contribute to overweight and obesity if consumed in excess.

Junk Foods

"Junk food" such as chips, candy bars, cakes, and cookies can be consumed in small quantities and limited to just rare occasions. Junk foods are readily available in today's world and, for the most part, taste good and are part of social gatherings. Therefore, truly avoiding these foods altogether is not realistic, so consuming them in moderation is the next best option. Allowing a small amount of these fun foods will teach children how to indulge responsibly in the future. After all, who doesn't like a piece of cake once in a while? In fact, this is the theme of this entire book—learning how to balance the enjoyment of food with responsible food choices.

Soda, however, can add many empty calories each day and should be severely limited or avoided. Children should be encouraged to substitute water, "diet" soda, "diet" lemonade, or an increasingly available array of flavored waters, which, typically, provide zero to one calorie per ounce, in place of regular soda. Low-calorie flavored low-fat milks and liquid yogurt-based drinks, generally 80 to 100 calories per 6 to 8 ounce serving, can add dietary calcium and protein as they quench thirst. Fruit juice is also a better choice than soda because it contains vitamins, but again excess consumption can lead to overweight. The American Academy of Pediatrics recommends that fruit juice be limited to 4 to 6 ounces daily for children between the ages of one and six. Children between seven and eighteen years old should not consume more than 8 to 12 ounces daily. Of course, the cheapest and best beverage is water!

How Many Calories Do Children and Adolescents Need?

Children and adolescents must consume enough calories to optimize health, promote growth and physical maturation, and support physical activity. Taking calories in excess of this amount can lead to overweight and obesity. When too few calories are consumed, new cells and tissues cannot be made and growth may be impaired.

The Estimated Energy Requirement (EER) is defined as the average amount of calories that are necessary to maintain energy balance in a healthy individual of a defined age, gender, height, and activity level. In children, this calculation must also include the energy needed to grow. Table 1 summarizes the EERs for children and adolescents.

How Much Protein Should Children and Adolescents Consume?

Protein deficiency in this country is very rare. Most American children consume protein in excess of the Recommended Dietary Allowance (RDA; the daily intake necessary to meet the nutritional requirements of 97–98 percent of the population). However, if energy intake is insufficient for any reason, dietary protein may be burned for energy, and as a result, body growth may suffer. This is true of adolescents with certain eating disorders. On the other hand, some young people try to gain strength and muscle mass by overconsuming protein. This practice can also be harmful since it can lead to dehydration and kidney damage. For most healthy children and adolescents, there is little reason to exceed the RDAs outlined in table 2.

Nutritional Problems: Eating Disorders, Obesity, and Chronic Diseases

Children and adolescents should be evaluated annually by a board certified pediatrician to ensure that growth, cognitive development, and sexual maturation are progressing as expected. When these parameters vary from the norm, a pediatrician will investigate.

Without question, the most pressing nutritional problem in pediatric offices across America is overweight and obesity. A pediatrician will not use the term *obese,* but instead will use such terms as *at risk for overweight* and *overweight* (see table 3). This is not meant to minimize the health impact of excess fat mass; rather, it is intended to encourage young people to lose weight without inflicting the emotional damage and stigma of the word *obese.* The fact remains that about one-third of obese adults were overweight as children. Perhaps more alarming is that a history of being overweight in childhood that persists into adulthood carries a greater risk of obesity-related complications (see table 4). Thus, intervening at the youngest age possible is vital to reversing the epidemic of obesity in America.

The emphasis placed on obesity in the last several years has certainly eclipsed other life-threatening nutritional disorders like "anorexia nervosa," or "anorexia" for short. Anorexia is a psychiatric disease characterized by low body weight and a body image distortion with an obsessive fear of gaining weight. About 0.3 percent of the population suffers from the disease, but 40 percent of all cases affect females between the ages of fifteen and nineteen years of age. Males are not spared. About 10 percent of individuals suffering from anorexia are male. Anorexia remains the psychiatric disorder with the highest mortality. Ten percent of individuals with anorexia eventually die of the disease. Less than 50 percent will have a lasting remission. Anorexia nervosa is a devastating disease that requires treatment from a team of many experts, including psychologists and medical doctors. A BMI of less than the 5th percentile for age should raise questions about the possibility of this disorder (see table 3).

Finally, there are a number of intestinal disorders (like celiac disease and inflammatory bowel disease; see chapter 4.5, "Nutrition and Digestive Problems") and other chronic diseases (like cystic fibrosis and congenital heart disease) that may predispose to malnutrition by malabsorption of calories and other nutrients or by a dramatic increase in energy requirements. These disorders may present with clear symptoms or as a subtle decline in weight or linear growth. This emphasizes the role of an annual examination by a pediatrician.

Conclusions

A calorie is a unit of energy, and energy is required to grow and to thrive. As one would put premium fuel in a fancy car, it is important that children are provided with the healthiest sources of energy available. Fruits, vegetables, whole grains, lean meats, fat-free dairy products, and healthy oils are the "premium" fuel that children and adolescents need to grow. Limiting television watching and computer time is as important as healthy eating. Children learn from parents and other adult role models. Thus, adults must lead by example. So, let's all *eat up* (healthy foods), *turn off* (computers and televisions), and *get out* (to walk and run)!

Table 1. Estimated Energy Requirements for Children and Adolescents.	
Children, 12-36 months (same equation for both genders): (89 x weight (kg) – 100) + 20 kcal For instance, a 12 kg 2 year old requires about: (89 x 12 – 100) + 20 = 988 kilocalories per day	
Boys	**Girls**
3-8 years 88.5 – (61.9 x age [y] + PA x (26.7 x weight [kg] + 903 x height [m]) + 20	3-8 years 135.3 – (30.8 x age [y]) x PA x (10.0 x weight [kg] + 934 x height [m]) + 20
9-18 years 88.5 – (61.9 x age [y]) + PA x (26.7 x weight [kg] + 903 x height [m]) = 25	9-18 years 135.3 – (30.8 x age [y]) + PA x (10.0 x weight [kg] +934 x height [m]) + 25
PA is an activity coefficient. For boys and girls aged 3-8 and boys aged 9-18. PA = 1.00 if child is sedentary PA = 1.13 if child is somewhat active PA = 1.26 if child is active PA = 1.42 if child is very active For girls aged 9-18 PA = 1.00 if child is sedentary PA = 1.16 if child is somewhat active PA = 1.31 if child is active PA = 1.56 if child is very active	
Dietary Reference Intakes for Energy, Carbohydrate, Fiber, Fat, Fatty Acids, Cholesterol, Protein, and Amino Acids. Institute of Medicine of the National Academies. The National Academies Press. Washington, D.C. 2005.	

Table 2. Recommended Daily Allowance of Protein for Children and Adolescents	
Boys and Girls	**RDA**
1 – 3 years	**1.05 grams/ kg/ day or 13 grams/ day**
4 – 8 years	**0.95 grams/ kg/ day or 19 grams/ day**
9 – 13 years	**0.95 grams/ kg/ day or 34 grams/ day**
Boys	**RDA**
14 – 18 years	**0.85 grams/ kg/ day or 52 grams/day**
Girls	**RDA**
14 – 18 years	**0.85 grams/ kg/ day or 46 grams/ day**
Dietary Reference Intakes for Energy, Carbohydrate, Fiber, Fat, Fatty Acids, Cholesterol, Protein, and Amino Acids. Institute of Medicine of the National Academies. The National Academies Press. Washington, D.C. 2005.	

Table 3. BMI (Body Mass Index = Weight in kilograms / Height in meters squared) Classifications in Childhood	
Classification	BMI
Underweight	BMI for age < 5th%
Healthy	BMI for age 5th % to 85th %
At risk of overweight	BMI for age 85th % to < 95%
Overweight	BMI for age > 95th%

Table 4. Complications of Obesity	
Diabetes Mellitus Type 2	Possible increased risk of cancer
High blood pressure	Arthritis
Stroke	Depressive symptoms
Heart disease	Gallbladder disease
Elevated bad cholesterol and triglycerides	Fatty liver
Obstructive sleep apnea	

Suggested Readings

AACE Power of Prevention. "Nutrition." http://www.powerofprevention.com/nutrition.php (accessed on September 30, 2008).

About.com. "Pediatrics: Nutrition for Children." http://pediatrics.about.com/od/nutrition/Nutrition_for_Children.htm (accessed on September 30, 2008).

American Heart Association. "Children and Nutrition." http://www.americanheart.org/presenter.jhtml?identifier=3007590 (accessed on September 22, 2008).

KeepKidsHealthy.com. "Children's nutrition guide." http://www.keepkidshealthy.com/nutrition/ (accessed on September 30, 2008).

Chapter 3.3

Women, Weight, and the Life Cycle: Maximizing Health by Minimizing Midlife Weight Gain

Harriette Mogul, MD

Weight gain in the middle decades of life represents a time-honored prophecy. Expanded waistlines are one of the least desirable and most predictable attributes of the mature woman. The appearance of excess pounds with each decade is well documented. Midlife weight gain (weight gain in the thirties and forties) was first highlighted in the early 1990s in a series of very important scientific publications from the "Nurses' Health Study," the nation's largest ongoing research study of women. Information from these studies clearly showed that the risk of developing diabetes, heart disease, breast cancer, and death from all causes increased with weight gain. Subsequent research has focused on the possible reasons for this connection between weight gain and disease as well as ways to prevent these problems. This chapter will summarize what is known about weight in midlife women and focus on recommendations to prevent weight gain and promote health during this important transition.

Midlife Weight Gain in the New Millennium

Weight trends in the United States demonstrate that women have higher rates of overweight and obesity than men. Overweight and obesity are seen mostly in adults aged forty to fifty-nine with even higher numbers of overweight and obesity among minority Americans in this age range. Information from a recent health survey (2003–2004) indicates that 88 percent of non-Hispanic black women and 80 percent of Mexican-American women aged forty to fifty-nine are overweight or obese (compared to 74 percent and 69 percent of women in the twenty- to thirty-nine-year-old groups). These trends provide a compelling argument for the need for intervention for women in this critical age range.

Why Women? Is Biology Destiny?

There is a wide range of potential explanations for midlife weight gain in women.

- Weight gain is an unexpected dividend of both shared living ("cohabitation") and pregnancy, as shown in many research studies.
- Women are the acknowledged caregivers for family members of all generations. Their designation as the sandwich generation aptly describes their roles as parents, partners,

and providers of care for older family folk. More than 50 percent of women work in full-time jobs, further diminishing time for exercise and dietary vigilance.

- Women biologically have slower basal metabolic rates than men, meaning their bodies burn fewer calories per day unrelated to physical activity.
- Women can have metabolic disturbances that contribute to weight gain, including:

1. *Disorders of the thyroid gland*

Women have higher rates of thyroid abnormalities, including hypothyroidism, than men. Hypothyroidism is a well-known cause of weight gain. The nonspecific nature of early symptoms of thyroid deficiency and the fact that many women in this age range do not seek regular medical care may delay the diagnosis and treatment of hypothyroidism in women. Hypothyroidism can be easily excluded by a simple blood test called "TSH," or "thyroid-stimulating hormone."

2. *The female hormones*

The decline of estrogen, progesterone, and other related hormones that start in the fifth decade are believed to be a factor in midlife weight gain. Definitive data have not yet established specific mechanisms that underlie the association between hormonal decline and weight gain in women. However, there is currently no evidence that estrogen or progesterone replacement minimizes this weight gain.

3. *Insulin resistance*

Some researchers suggest that insulin resistance and insulin elevations may be associated with progressive refractory weight gain in distinct female subpopulations. It is well known that insulin resistance tends to worsen with age.

4. *Prescription medications*

Women have high rates of several underlying disorders that increase the use of medications that cause weight gain. Depression is a notable example. Women have higher rates of depression at all ages than men—with a lifetime prevalence rate of 20 percent. They are also more likely to seek treatment for symptoms of depression from primary care and specialty physicians. Many of the most widely prescribed antidepressants, the SSRIs ("selective serotonin reuptake inhibitors"), cause weight gain and are typically used long-term. The decline of estrogen replacement for symptoms relating to the menopausal transition and the approval of SSRIs for treatment of these symptoms further increase the use of these medications by midlife women. Weight should be carefully monitored in women following the initiation of treatment with antidepressants and other medications (such as antihistamines) known to cause weight gain.

Prevention and Predictors: Lessons from the First Wave of Studies

Prevention of midlife weight gain in women has been the focus of several large research studies. The first, the "Power of Prevention Study," evaluated the impact of two "low intensity" interventions on weight gain in adults aged twenty to forty-five (80 percent of whom were female). Despite educational materials encouraging weight monitoring; increased physical activity, especially walking; and dietary changes (increased fruits and vegetables and decreased fat), 63 percent of participants gained weight in the three-year study period. Another research study, called the "Women's Healthy Lifestyle Project," of 535 women aged forty-four to fifty who did not have menopause by the time of the study showed less weight gain with a low-calorie, low-fat diet and exercise compared with a group of women who continued their usual lifestyle. However, the summary report raised concerns about how effective weight gain prevention programs can actually be. The researchers concluded that "weight gain prevention is a challenging task [and] novel approaches to the prevention of weight gain are needed."

The Focus on Fat and Fiber: Long-term Research Studies

Mounting concerns over the increase in childhood and adult obesity have produced several large studies looking at the role of fat, fiber, fruits, and vegetables in promoting weight loss or preventing weight gain. One of these research studies, the CARDIA study, was a ten-year multi-center study of several thousand young adults, ages eighteen to thirty years, with 53 percent being women. This study found that fiber consumption was more strongly related to weight gain and insulin levels than fat. The study also found that "high fiber diets may protect against obesity…by lowering insulin levels."

Another large research study, the Women's Health Initiative (or the "WHI") Dietary Modification Trial, looked at 50,000 postmenopausal women. In this study, the intervention was weekly dietary counseling sessions aimed at reducing total fat intake to 20 percent and increasing the intake of fruit, vegetables, and fiber. This intervention produced greater weight loss than those women not receiving the intervention. It was particularly exciting that the weight loss could be maintained for an average of 7 ½ years. In this study, weight loss was greatest among women in both groups who decreased their fat intake and increased vegetable and fruit servings without a significant effect of increased dietary fiber. This is contrary to what many people thought would happen since the calories in low-fat diets can be more than made up for with high-calorie starchy foods. Nevertheless, this study concluded that a *low-fat* eating pattern does *not* result in weight gain in postmenopausal women.

While the goals, methods, and findings of these two long-term studies are not directly related, taken together they support the importance of increasing fruits and vegetables in long-term maintenance of weight, as reflected in earlier studies.

The Case for Calcium

The importance of calcium for bone health is well recognized and forms one of the earliest nutrition lessons learned in childhood. However, the big news about calcium is not about bones; it is about body weight. Researchers are taking a new look at calcium. One of the most interesting early findings, now shown in more than one research study, is the association between high dietary calcium intake and a slowing down of weight gain in many different age groups. While still controversial, many experts now suggest that dietary calcium may play an important role in weight regulation.

The relationship between dietary calcium, weight, and even the risk of insulin resistance, one of the key problems in diabetes, has been a topic of intense research in the past decade. As first shown in the National Health and Nutrition Examination Study (or "NHANES"), the largest ongoing US study of health and nutrition trends across the nation, people with the highest intake of calcium and dairy products had the lowest level of obesity. Subsequent studies confirmed these findings in children, men, and some, but not all, studies of women.

Support for the regulation of weight by dietary calcium and mechanisms that underlie this relationship have been demonstrated in an increasing number of laboratory studies. Several clinical studies have also assessed the role of dietary and supplemental calcium in weight regulation. These include short-term weight reduction trials (of both women and men) and long-term dietary studies of large populations of postmenopausal women. The WHI (described above) studied the effect of supplemental calcium, given as 1,000 milligrams per day plus 400 units of vitamin D, on weight gain in over 36,000 women. This study showed that calcium plus vitamin D had a small but consistently favorable effect on preventing weight gain, which was observed primarily in women who had inadequate calcium intake before they started the study.

Several calcium intervention trials have yielded contradictory findings. As with other controversial conclusions from well-designed research studies, some of the differences in these findings can be explained by differences in the study populations. Nevertheless, when taken together, the various intervention studies suggest that increasing dietary calcium may be most beneficial in midlife women who are overweight, obese, or have diabetes. This is best accomplished by substituting calcium-rich foods for other foods without increasing the total number of calories. In summary:

- high dietary calcium intake is associated with weight loss,
- increasing dietary calcium intake could substantially reduce the risk of overweight, and
- the anti-obesity effect is greater with dairy calcium than supplemental sources.

Fortunately, there are now many ways to add low-calorie, low-fat dairy products to the diet. Here are a few suggestions:

1. Low-fat yogurt is available in 6- and 8-ounce containers that typically range from 60 to 150 calories and provide 245 to 384 milligrams of calcium. These can be purchased in bulk in big-box stores and are frequently on sale at supermarkets, making them affordable for most American households. Adding seasonal fruits, such as berries, creates a healthy, convenient, and transportable breakfast.
2. Yogurt "smoothies" or fruit milkshakes can be made by blending 8 ounces (1 cup) of low-fat yogurt and/or milk with 1 cup of fresh or frozen fruit to provide nearly 300 milligrams of calcium. This can be assembled in the container of a blender or a food processor in the evening to make breakfast preparation easier. One or two teaspoons of honey can be added for additional sweetness if needed.
3. Low-fat lattes can be purchased at a number of national coffee chains and generally provide 300 milligrams of calcium per serving. These are available plain in caffeinated and decaffeinated versions and can be flavored with sugar-free syrups, like vanilla, hazelnut, and dulce de leche.

4. Low-fat cottage cheese provides 137 milligrams of calcium per cup. Cottage cheese can be eaten along with fresh or water-packed fruit or whole-grain toast for a healthy breakfast.
5. Low-fat feta cheese, low-fat mozzarella cheese, and other reduced-fat cheeses provide approximately 275 to 300 milligrams of calcium per 1 ½ ounces and make excellent choices for meals and snacks.
6. "Cream" soups can be made by pureeing fresh or frozen chopped or diced vegetables (carrots, cauliflower, peas, squash, spinach, etc.) and then cooking in vegetable (or low-sodium chicken) stock with low-fat milk (for warm soup) or low-fat yogurt (for cold soup). Try seasoning to taste with curry powder, ginger (powdered or freshly grated), or fresh or dried herbs.
7. No-sugar-added low-fat prepared puddings are available and range from 80 to 110 calories per serving. These provide approximately 100 milligrams of calcium per cup.
8. Frozen yogurt; low-fat, no-sugar-added ice cream bars; and other single-serving low-calorie ice cream products are filling the frozen food section shelves in supermarkets across the country. At 100 to 140 calories per serving, these are great low-calorie substitutes for the usual high-calorie, high-fat versions and add variety to the diet, in addition to serving as a source of dietary calcium providing approximately 90 to 100 milligrams of calcium per ½ cup.
9. Fat-free hot cocoa mixes containing 300 milligrams of calcium (the same as in a cup of milk) and only 50 calories per serving are another excellent source of dietary calcium.

Integrating Exercise

Studies show that regular aerobic exercise maintains weight loss and prevents weight regain in women. However, many midlife women find it difficult to add exercise to their busy lives. Sedentary lifestyle is a characteristic of large percentages of American women and is independent of socioeconomic status. Recent studies suggest that even brief periods of exercise (for example, in blocks of fifteen minutes) add up and can provide benefits when done regularly. Women with otherwise insufficient time to exercise at a gym can start by adding one or two fifteen-minute segments of an exercise routine or brisk walk each day. This can be particularly useful for the "de-conditioned," midlife woman. The following sections will provide a few examples of physical activities that can be integrated into a healthy lifestyle.

The Home Exercise Studio

Women who prefer to exercise at home can rent or purchase exercise videotapes or DVDs, widely available since Jane Fonda first introduced a generation of midlife women to the benefits of home exercise more than two decades ago. Women's magazines contain new articles each month with glossy views demonstrating the correct technique for strength training, as well as improving coordination and balance. As a general rule, women should start slowly and work up gradually. Low-cost exercise aids that include rubber resistance bands; hand weights in one-, two- and five-pound weight ranges; and exercise balls, now available in many drug stores and supermarkets, as well as big-box and home stores, can enhance these exercise routines.

Walking

For women in safe urban, suburban, and rural settings, walking can provide relaxation along with all other benefits of regular exercise, such as improved heart health. Working women in similar settings can use part of their lunchtime breaks to incorporate a brisk twenty- to forty-minute walk in the company of others or the privacy of their MP3 players. For some women, even walking to or home from work may be an option.

Dancing

Dancing is an underappreciated and fun-filled way to increase caloric expenditure. Dance is an important element of many cultures worldwide. Ballroom dancing, folk dancing, and simply moving to music to pick up the pace while performing household chores count as exercise.

Summary

In summary, the promotion of weight loss and prevention of weight gain in midlife women remain important challenges. Specific strategies that address the time constraints, schedule demands, and responsibilities of midlife women are an important part of a healthy lifestyle that can improve longevity and the quality of life.

Selected Readings

American Dietetic Association. "Eat right: Nutrition and women's health." http://www.eatright.org/cps/rde/xchg/ada/hs.xsl/advocacy_3780_ENU_HTML.htm (accessed on October 24, 2008).

American Medical Women's Association. "Nutrition and women's health." http://www.amwa-doc.org/index.cfm?objectId=42C359DF-D567-0B25-5B5E787B474A3BDD (accessed on October 24, 2008).

Mogul H, Stafford D. Syndrome W: A woman's guide to reversing mid-life weight gain. M. Evans, 2005.

US Department of Health and Human Services. WomensHealth.gov. "Staying active and eating healthy." http://www.womenshealth.gov/FitnessNutrition/ (accessed on October 19, 2008).

US Food and Drug Administration. "Information for women on food safety, nutrition and cosmetics." http://www.cfsan.fda.gov/~dms/wh-toc.html (accessed on October 24, 2008).

Chapter 3.4

Nutritional Guidelines for Pregnancy

Carol Levy, MD

We have all heard the statement of "Eat more, you are eating for two" said to women who are pregnant. However, this statement often leads to the misconception that nutritional requirements of pregnant women are doubled. For most women, nutrient needs do increase during pregnancy and are necessary to ensure the development of a healthy baby. Eating a well-balanced diet is the best way to reach nutritional goals. Among the nutrients that deserve a special focus during pregnancy are protein, calcium, iron, folate, and adequate calories. In this chapter, these nutrients will be reviewed as well as the role of prenatal vitamins. Appropriate weight gain will be discussed based on current guidelines. Special circumstances including nausea and vomiting, gestational diabetes, "hypoglycemia," and breast-feeding will also be reviewed.

Protein

Pregnant women need about an extra 25 grams of protein each day to support the expansion of the blood volume, uterus, and breasts. Protein choices should be ones with the greatest nutritional value. Chicken, lean cuts of beef, low-mercury fishes (see later), eggs, tofu, and low-fat dairy products are all good options. One ounce of meat is equal to 7 grams of protein. Typically, most pregnant women are able to meet this goal fairly easily. If a woman does not consume meat or dairy products, she may need to consult with a registered dietitian to help her attain her protein goals.

Calcium

The Recommended Dietary Allowance for calcium consumption during pregnancy is 1,000 milligrams. When a woman is having trouble reaching this goal, a calcium supplement is often recommended. Consuming calcium during pregnancy helps to ensure the mother's bone mass is preserved as the baby's skeleton develops. Early in pregnancy, intestinal absorption of calcium is doubled, and the mineral is stored in the mother's bones. During the third trimester, when the baby's skeletal growth peaks and teeth are being formed, the fetus draws about 300 milligrams each day of calcium from the mother. Dairy products such as milk, cheese, and yogurt as well as calcium-fortified orange juice are the most concentrated sources of dietary calcium. Other less calcium-rich options include dried beans, tofu, calcium-fortified soy milk, fish with tiny bones, and dark green leafy vegetables.

Iron

During pregnancy, the recommended intake for iron increases from 18 to 27 milligrams per day to meet the needs of both the mother and fetus. Meeting this increased need for iron is often difficult. Many women are already iron deficient when they become pregnant and are trying to make up for this. Iron-rich supplements, as well as foods rich in iron, are often recommended. Foods rich in iron include meat, dark poultry, cooked clams and oysters, legumes, and enriched grain products. Fruits rich in vitamin C can help enhance iron absorption.

Folic Acid

Folate and folic acid refer to the same water-soluble B-complex vitamin. Folate is found naturally in food, whereas folic acid is the salt form of folate found in dietary supplements, like multivitamins. In this chapter, we will use the term *folic acid* to refer to this vitamin. A pregnant woman's need for folic acid is 50 percent greater than that of a non-pregnant woman. The current Recommended Dietary Allowance for pregnancy is 600 micrograms of folic acid. Research has shown that adequate folic acid intake in pregnancy may be associated with a reduction in neural tube defects. The major sources of folic acid in the diet are green leafy vegetables, liver, citrus fruits, juices, as well as fortified grains and cereals. For women planning to become pregnant, folic acid supplementation is recommended through a multivitamin to ensure that intake is adequate.

Iodine

Recent studies suggest that iodine deficiency during pregnancy can affect both maternal and infant thyroid function as well as cognitive development of the infant. Although currently there is currently a lack of clinical data on the effect of iodine deficiency and birth outcomes in women with mild to moderate iodine deficiency, several health authorities currently recommend pregnant women consume 150mcg of potassium iodide daily. Some dietary sources of iodine include iodized salt, milk, fortified breads and cereals, and seaweed. Caution should be used in obtaining supplements from seaweed or kelp supplements, as content can be variable and sometimes lead to toxic levels. Check with your healthcare provider as to what would be best for you and check the labeling on your prenatal vitamin, as many are not fortified.

Foods to Eat with Caution during Pregnancy

Although dietary restrictions and recommendations for specific foods should be discussed with a patient's physician, there are specific warnings with regard to fish that address a specific type of infection, called "listeriosis." Listeriosis is a harmful bacterial infection that can be transmitted to the unborn baby even if the mother shows no signs of infection. Listeriosis can also be found in some ready-to-eat refrigerated foods and unpasteurized dairy products. Luncheon meats, hot dogs, pâtés, meat spreads, and unpasteurized cheese should be avoided.

Fish are generally a good source of lean protein consumption, and some of the fattier varieties provide excellent sources of DHA and EPA (docosahexaenoic acid and eicosapentanoic acid; two types of omega-3 fatty acids important for fetal brain and vision development; see chapter 2.2, "Fats"). Unfortunately, certain fish can also contain metals such as mercury, which can affect fetus brain development. Examples of fish to be avoided are shark, swordfish, king mackerel, and tilefish. Some forms of tuna (albacore) are also quite high in mercury. It is safe to consume up to 12 ounces of fish weekly. If individual weekly consumption is more in one particular week, it should then be reduced the following week. Since guidelines on this subject are continually changing, pregnant women should discuss fish intake and the risks of mercury exposure with their obstetricians.

Weight Gain and Caloric Intake

Caloric requirements for pregnancy are generally determined to be 300 kilocalories above standard caloric intake. Depending on a woman's pre-pregnancy weight, the caloric goals and recommended weight gain are often modified. So where does the weight go?

For women at their ideal body weight prior to pregnancy, a 25 to 35 pounds weight gain for the entire pregnancy is recommended. This generally correlates to a caloric consumption of 30 kilocalories for every kilogram of body weight prior to becoming pregnant. In order to calculate the body weight in kilograms, divide the body weight in pounds by 2.2 (so a 121-pound woman weighs 55 kilograms). In terms of the optimal rate of weight gain during pregnancy, general recommendations are for a 2- to 4-pound weight gain in the first trimester (1–13 weeks). In the second (weeks 14–27) and third (weeks 28–40) trimesters of pregnancy, approximately a pound a week of weight gain is generally recommended. Women who are petite (less than 5 feet 2 inches) should target weight goals in the lower end of the range. It is also important to be aware that weight gain can fluctuate. Some weeks, only a half a pound may be added, and another week, more than a pound may be added.

Women with special circumstances may have different goals. Women who are underweight should consume 35 to 40 calories per kilogram body weight (or about 16–18 calories per pound body weight) for a goal of 28 to 40 pounds weight gain. Overweight women should target 25 calories per kilogram body weight (or about 11 calories per pound) for a 15 to 25-pound weight gain. Obese women are generally encouraged to set a goal of 11 to 20 pounds weight gain for the entire pregnancy. Twin pregnancies should target a 35 to 45-pound weight gain and triplet pregnancies, 45 to 50 pounds.

Risks associated with too little weight gain for pregnancy are low birth weight babies (less than 5.5 pounds) or very low birth weight babies (less than 3.5 pounds) as well as premature delivery. Risks of excessive weight gain include weight retention after delivery (the more you gain, the more you have to lose), "gestational diabetes," as well as pregnancy-induced hypertension (high blood pressure). In spite of the risks of pregnancy-induced obesity, weight loss diets are almost never recommended during pregnancy.

Nausea

Food cravings and food aversions are very common during pregnancy. They may also be associated with the common complaint of "morning sickness." Typically, symptoms are the worst during the first fifteen weeks of pregnancy but may persist for the duration of the pregnancy. Changing levels of a hormone called progesterone can affect the way food is emptied from the stomach. Rarely, medication may be required if severe vomiting and poor oral intake occurs. In extreme circumstances, patients may require hospitalization if they become dehydrated and require intravenous nutrition ("parenteral nutrition") to meet dietary goals. Some guidelines on specific food choices that can reduce nausea are listed below.

TYPE OF FOOD	RESPONSE	EXPLANATION
Meat	Increases nausea	Fat is difficult to digest
Carbohydrates	Reduced nausea	Simple carbohydrates reduce stomach acid and are easy to digest
Skim Milk	Reduced nausea	Fat can also slow down the digestive system and skim milk has no fat
Citrus fruits	Reduced nausea	Vitamin C content enhances digestion

Women also find that frequent small meals, plenty of sleep, and avoidance of certain smells can reduce nausea as well.

Gestational Diabetes

Diabetes discovered during pregnancy is called gestational diabetes. This condition is associated with blood sugar levels higher than what is considered normal during pregnancy. Risks of this condition include large babies (known as "macrosomia"), premature deliveries, low blood sugar ("hypoglycemia") in the baby at delivery, delayed maturation of the fetus's lungs, and a weaker placenta. Most pregnant women will undergo testing of the way their bodies handle large amounts of carbohydrate while they are pregnant. Generally, this occurs between twenty-four and twenty-eight weeks of pregnancy but may occur earlier in patients felt to be at higher risk (family history of diabetes, obesity, known prior pregnancy with gestational diabetes, or polycystic ovary syndrome [PCOS]). Hormones produced during pregnancy lead to "insulin resistance." In this state, pregnant women will not respond as well to insulin, making it more difficult to keep the blood sugar level in the normal range.

One of the most important features for managing gestational diabetes is controlling the amount of carbohydrate eaten with each meal. Too much carbohydrate will lead to elevations in glucose levels. Generally speaking, dietary guidelines include smaller consumption of starches at meals, smaller meals with snacks, higher fiber (such as whole grain) carbohydrate choices, and avoidance of juices or sugar-containing beverages. Meal planning is done on an individual basis. In addition, blood glucose testing is needed to ensure a woman's blood glucose levels remain in the desired range. Based on a woman's pre-pregnancy and current pregnancy weight, weight gain goals may be modified. Women with gestational diabetes are often counseled by a registered dietitian or diabetes educator.

After delivery and the loss of pregnancy weight, a goal of reaching a healthy body weight should be discussed with the physician. Having had gestational diabetes during pregnancy increases the risk of the mother developing diabetes in the future, especially with subsequent pregnancies.

Hypoglycemia

Women can often feel lightheaded or faint during pregnancy due to shifts in blood pressure and dehydration. At times, these symptoms might be incorrectly attributed to true hypoglycemia since the blood sugar tests might not actually be abnormally low. In fact, blood sugars in pregnancy can normally be in the high 50s to low 60s. Dizziness and lightheadedness from hunger can also make a pregnant woman feel unwell. Frequent snacks and adequate hydration will almost always remedy these symptoms. True hypoglycemia can occur in pregnant women with diabetes if meals are missed and the patient is taking medications like insulin that can lower glucose levels.

Breast-feeding

Breast-feeding is encouraged for all women after delivery. A woman's calorie, fluid, protein, vitamin, and mineral requirements are increased while breast-feeding. When a woman is breast-feeding, or lactating, she must meet her own nutritional needs as well as produce an adequate amount of milk to meet her baby's needs. Caloric needs for lactation are typically increased by 330 calories each day for the first six months and by 400 calories each day during the second six months. Calcium intake should be targeted at 1,000 milligrams each day. Certain foods may need to be avoided if the baby does not seem to tolerate those foods in the mother's diet. Diets providing less than 1,800 calories each day are not recommended.

Summary

Pregnancy is an exciting time for women but can also be associated with some confusion about nutrition. Adequate and appropriate nutrient intake will ensure the best outcomes for both the mother and baby. Working with a physician and a registered dietitian, when needed, will help mothers achieve this goal.

Suggested Readings

American Diabetes Association. *Medical management of pregnancy complicated by diabetes, Third Edition.* ADA, Alexandria, VA, 2000.

American Pregnancy Association. http://www.americanpregnancy.org/pregnancyhealth/pregnancynutrition.html (accessed on October 18, 2008).

MayoClinic.com. "Essential nutrients when you are eating for two." http://www.mayoclinic.com/health/pregnancy-nutrition/PR00110 (accessed on October 18, 2008).

MayoClinic.com. "Healthy eating for you and your baby." http://www.mayoclinic.com/health/pregnancy-nutrition/PR00108 (accessed on October 18, 2008).

MayoClinic.com. "Pregnancy nutrition: Foods to avoid." http://www.mayoclinic.com/health/pregnancy-nutrition/PR00109 (accessed on October 18, 2008).

The Ohio State University. "Nutritional needs of pregnancy." http://ohioline.osu.edu/mob-fact/0001.html (accessed on October 18, 2008).

Chapter 3.5

Nutrition for Men

Ronald Tamler, MD, PhD, MBA, CNSP

All human beings have similar bodily functions, but, indeed, there are also many biochemical and physiological differences between men and women. These differences account for the special medical needs that men have. Among these medical needs are, of course, some special nutritional needs.

Men die on average six years earlier than women, and they are more likely to die from heart attack, stroke, diabetes, and cancer. Men are less likely to take care of themselves than women. They are less likely to have health insurance, seek out doctors to prevent disease, and eat right, and they tend to work in more dangerous jobs than women. While most rules and guidelines regarding nutrition and physical activity that apply to women are also true for men, this chapter deals with special concerns. . .just for men!

Men and Obesity

Many of us are overweight or obese. If your body mass index (see chapter 4.2, "Nutrition and Obesity") is 25 or greater, then you are overweight, and if it is 30 or greater, then you are obese. Try a little experiment: check your waist circumference. Take a tape measure and hold the beginning to your belly button. Then find out how far the tape measure stretches to wrap around you to get back to your belly button. If it is more than 40 inches (even less if you are Asian), your waist circumference is too high. This means that you have a lot of fat tissue in your belly. Not all fat tissue is created equal, and the fat in your belly, called "visceral fat," has the greatest effect on your health. It has adverse effects on your blood vessels and your hormones.

Obese men have a much higher risk of high blood pressure, heart attack, stroke, and certain cancers. They also tend to have trouble with their joints, as they have to carry all the weight. Another problem is "obstructive sleep apnea." In this condition, men start to snore and eventually stop breathing for brief periods at a time during their sleep. This breathing problem usually gets better when men lose weight, as does the risk for heart attack and stroke.

Obesity and Hormones in Men

Most people have heard of the male hormone "testosterone." It works on many levels: testosterone makes muscles strong and makes body hair grow; it helps the brain; it strengthens bones; and it gives men lots of energy and sexual drive. Fat tissue has a special enzyme called "aromatase." As obese men gain more and more weight, their fat tissue whisks away testosterone and, by using aromatase, turns it into the female hormone, estrogen. This is especially the case with the fat in the belly. Not only is there less testosterone left, but the estrogen also sends a signal to the body to make less testosterone. The result is decreased sex drive and even reduced erectile function, or "impotence." Another result of decreased testosterone and increased estrogen is breast growth, called "gynecomastia." Finally, the number and the quality of sperm that men produced is dramatically decreased in obese men.

Is there something that can be done for this? There sure is. Many studies have shown over and over again that weight loss leads to higher testosterone levels, better sex drive, and improved erections. Even a weight loss of 5 to 10 percent can lead to improved results. Interestingly, men who undergo weight-loss surgery (called "bariatric surgery") tend to have a similar experience. However, the connection between testosterone and obesity works both ways. Men with low testosterone tend to gain more weight from fat over the years.

Underweight and Hormones in Men

Men with unusually low weight, such as people with HIV/AIDS, cancer, or eating disorders also have trouble with low testosterone levels, with similarly bad sexual drive and impotence. In addition, they tend to have weaker bones. It appears that the sweet spot for men, when it comes to sexual function and weight, is simply a normal weight with a normal BMI.

Nutrition and Sexual Function in Men

There is a difference between sexual drive, also called "libido," and erectile function, also called "potency." Sexual drive comes from the brain and is influenced by many things, among them testosterone. Potency is the ability of the penis to stay rigid as long as it needs to in order to have sexual intercourse successfully. It is influenced mainly by how healthy the blood vessels are, but testosterone also plays a role.

As men age and usually gain weight, both aspects of sexual function get worse. Men have tried for thousands of years to improve matters with special foods. Starfish were sold as aphrodisiacs on the streets of ancient Rome; potable gold was heralded as the path to sexual prowess in medieval times; and even the biblical King David suffered from impotence, though it is not certain what remedies he tried. Other foods with supposed effects on libido and impotence are celery, caviar, and even the testicles of various animals, sometimes referred to as "mountain oysters." The bottom line for folk remedies seems to be that "if it tastes good, if it's not harmful," and "if you believe in it, nothing bad will happen" (except to the wallet if one overdoes the caviar).

Most studies with medications for impotence show a placebo effect in 25 percent of the participants. This means that 25 percent who were taking a sugar pill felt their impotence was getting better.

There are certain nutritional supplements that promise improvement and have been studied for impotence. The oldest one is "yohimbine," an extract from tree bark that works on the blood vessels of the penis. It works for mild impotence, but its effectiveness and safety are not as good as established medications that target impotence. Another supplement that is available is called

"DHEA" (which is an abbreviation for "dehydroepiandrosterone"), a hormone that is made in the adrenal gland. DHEA can be turned into testosterone in the body, but it really does not do much for sex drive or potency most of the time. "L-Arginine" is an amino acid that can help the blood vessels in the penis, and it works better when combined with yohimbine, or the maritime pine bark extract "pycnogenol." It is important to note that impotence might be an early sign of future heart problems, so you should tell your doctor if you are experiencing problems.

Nutrition for Prostate Health

There are two issues regarding the prostate that men can face. First, there can be an enlargement of the prostate with advancing age, which is not due to cancer, called "benign prostatic hyperplasia" (BPH). The growing prostate wraps around the tube that leads the urine from the bladder out of the body (called the "urethra"). When this enlargement is too much, it may result in trouble with urination. Men with BPH can experience increased straining with urination, dribbling, urge to urinate, and frequent urination, which can interrupt normal sleep at night. "Saw palmetto," the extract of the American dwarf palm tree, has been shown to improve symptoms in research studies. In fact, many research studies show that it works just as well as regular drugs, although nobody knows why. Certain pumpkin seeds may also work, but there is not as much literature to confirm their efficacy.

Another great challenge for men as they age is prostate cancer. Every year, 230,000 men will be diagnosed with prostate cancer and about 30,000 will die of it. It is not surprising that many men try to use nutrition to decrease their odds of getting prostate cancer. "Lycopene," an antioxidant found in red tomatoes, can have a good effect on preventing prostate cancer. Interestingly, the effect is better with cooked and pureed tomatoes, so keep that pasta sauce close (just don't overeat on the pasta). Another category of remedies are "polyphenols" and "flavonoids." These are also antioxidants that are found in fruit, vegetables, red wine, and tea, and are often marketed as extracts of grape seed or green tea. The jury is still out regarding alcohol for preventing prostate cancer. One study found a 6 percent reduction of risk for every glass of red wine per week, but another study found better results with beer. However, excessive alcohol drinking will not benefit prostate health and may lead to weight gain, serious health problems, motor vehicle accidents, and alcoholism.

Tea, especially green tea, contains polyphenols with very strong antioxidant properties and may decrease the risk of prostate cancer, but it can also be harmful if one drinks too much of it. Pomegranate juice may be effective not just in reducing the risk for prostate cancer but also reducing the progression of prostate cancer once it is diagnosed. Soy contains other substances that affect how male and female hormones are made and how they work. Several studies have shown that people who eat more soy have less prostate cancer. However, one cannot have it all. Soy and other plant foods, such as beer, contain "phytoestrogens." These plant products work in the body like the female hormone, estrogen. Therefore, the overuse of phytoestrogens takes us full circle to the beginning of this chapter with the adverse effects of too much estrogen in men.

In summary, although various dietary supplements and foods have been studied and found to have properties associated with improvement in medical conditions, they are not a replacement for seeing a doctor and taking conventional medical therapies when recommended.

Selected Reading

Barnard R. Prostate cancer prevention by nutritional means to alleviate metabolic syndrome. Am J Clin Nutr, 2007 Sep; 86(3):s889-93.

Esposito K, Giugliano F, Di Palo C, et al. Effect of lifestyle changes on erectile dysfunction in obese men: A randomized controlled trial. JAMA 2004 Jun 23; 291(24):2978-84.

Niskanen L, Laaksonen D, Punnonen K, et al. Changes in sex hormone-binding globulin and testosterone during weight loss and weight maintenance in abdominally obese men with the metabolic syndrome. Diabetes, Obes Metab 2004 May; 6(3):208-15.

Tamler R, Mechanick J. Dietary supplements and nutraceuticals in the management of andrologic disorders._Endocrinol Metab Clin North Am 2007 Jun; 36(2):533-52.

Chapter 3.6

Nutrition for the Elderly

Yi-Hao Yu, MD, PhD, FACE, CNSP

The elderly are a unique subpopulation with respect to nutritional care. The Merriam-Webster Dictionary defines *elderly* as people who are older than "middle age." However, the age cutoff for the elderly varies over time and in different countries. Being elderly is often associated with being at the retirement age or the age at which one can begin to receive pension benefits. Some developing countries use age fifty or fifty-five as a cutoff for the elderly, whereas most Western countries accept sixty or sixty-five to define the elderly. It is clear, then, that the age cutoff for the elderly is somewhat arbitrary.

Regardless of whether one's age falls into the "elderly" category by definition, one should know how age itself can affect proper nutrition. Obviously, biological age (true age) is important, but physiological age (reflected by overall health and aging status) is even more relevant. This is because nutritional needs are related to various health conditions, physical activity levels, and medical and surgical histories.

Since the elderly encompass a wide age span and are a group of variable health status, there is no one-size-fits-all strategy for meeting their nutritional needs and goals. However, there are still commonalities among people in this diverse age group. In general, because of aging, the elderly are more vulnerable to malnutrition, either "overnutrition" or "undernutrition." On one hand, aging makes people more susceptible to metabolic diseases like diabetes, heart disease, cancer, and several other chronic diseases. The risk for these diseases increases with overweight and obesity. On the other hand, the elderly are also particularly vulnerable to undernutrition due to various causes.

Age-related Loss of Muscle Mass

One of the most noticeable changes in body composition with age is the loss of skeletal muscle mass and strength. This phenomenon is referred to as "sarcopenia." Accompanied by the loss of muscle mass is the relative increase in body fat. This is particularly true for the fat in the abdomen, which is sometimes referred to as "central adiposity." *Marked central adiposity*, or *central obesity*, is a term that may be used even in people who are not obese. In many elderly people, abdominal fat accumulation is very prominent, while their muscle mass in the limbs is actually quite small and their body weight is actually "normal."

In addition to developing sarcopenia, the elderly are more prone to become "frail." With significant frailty, elderly people can experience unexplained anorexia, weight loss, or body tissue wasting. This can be associated with severe physical, mental, and immune function problems. This overall condition is also referred to as "geriatric cachexia." Regardless of the label that is used for this debilitating state, it is still a very dire condition.

Age-related loss of muscle mass may begin as early as thirty years of age. More than 50 percent of muscle mass can be gradually lost by age eighty. Scientists are not completely certain about the extent to which other factors such as chronic diseases may contribute to this process, but aging plays a direct role. Aging causes hormonal changes, deterioration of the central and peripheral nervous system that connects and controls muscles, and decline in the contractility of muscle cells—all of which play a role in sarcopenia. The questions are: What are the consequences of loss of muscle mass, and how can this process be slowed or prevented?

Loss of muscle mass has at least three consequences. First, a reduction of muscle mass is associated with decreases in whole body energy expenditure and overall metabolism. This is because muscle is where the largest portion of the body's metabolism takes place. The decline in metabolism poses higher risks for sugar and fat intolerance, diabetes, and other metabolic and cardiovascular diseases. This is particularly true if the amount of calories consumed is more than what the body needs.

Second, a reduction of muscle mass leads to declines in physical capability and functional performance. This consequence is particularly bad because once a person's physical activity is affected and subsequently limited due to sarcopenia, a vicious cycle may ensue. As muscles are not used, muscle mass decreases, then the person is weaker and uses less muscle, and the cycle goes on and on. These events are easily observed in anyone suffering severe illness.

Third, muscle tissue is an important energy and amino acid reserve that can be called upon during illness. Amino acids are the building blocks for protein. Amino acids are liberated from muscle in response to various illness, trauma, injury, and inflammation. These amino acids can be used by the immune system to fight disease and by the liver to supply energy for the brain. In the intensive care unit, patients are usually unable to eat enough to maintain appropriate body functions. Therefore, elderly patients who start out with depleted lean body mass are simply at higher risk for dying in the hospital than elderly patients who are healthy and well-nourished before their hospitalization.

Despite the almost certain decline in muscle mass with aging, the pace and amount of the decline can be modified. A person can actually have some control over this aging process, but only with commitment and perseverance. Studies of physically active senior citizens and athletes in advanced ages support this idea. "Progressive resistance training" is a technique that can build up muscle strength and functional performance. The elderly should participate in not only activities such as walking and stair climbing, but also even a little weight lifting. This can be effectively accomplished even in frail nursing home residents who are in their seventies, eighties, and even nineties, as long as proper instruction and medical supervision are provided. These kinds of activities can preserve muscle mass, improve the immune system, and have overall benefits on organ function and well-being. So, the take-home message is to stay active and exercise regularly, no matter how old you are. It takes courage to keep exercising regularly, even if you do not feel like doing it. If regular exercise is done in order to increase total physical activity, one can prevent the downward-spiraling path towards accelerated aging and health deterioration.

What has sarcopenia to do with nutrition? With muscle mass loss and a decreased metabolic rate, fewer calories need to be consumed in order to maintain a healthy body weight. This adjustment in reducing food intake is often hard to do and is not without risk. Smaller meals can increase the risk for certain vitamin and mineral deficiencies. This means that the quality of a diet—types of foods and the nutritional values of protein—become as important as the quantity of a diet. As a rule of thumb, compared with a regular diet for young people, a diet for the elderly should contain relatively less fat, sugar, and starch, and more high-quality protein (lean meats, egg whites, dairy products, and beans). People with kidney problems should consult with a physician or registered dietitian to determine the right amount of protein for their diets.

Altered Sensory Function, Changes in Food Palatability, and Reduced Energy Intake

Another important change associated with aging is the decrease of appetite. This is called "anorexia." The cause of this is even more complex because in addition to biological changes, there are certain social, economical, and psychological factors that also affect the elderly. First, with reduced physical activity, the body may respond by not having an appetite for big meals. In a way, this is a healthy response because the body does not want to take in more food than it can handle. However, the body's regulatory system can sometimes misinterpret what is happening and fail to regulate appetite according to the body's energy needs. Social isolation, inability to shop for or prepare tasty meals because of physical limitation, and depression can all lead to poor appetite and undernutrition in the elderly. Medical or surgical illness may also have a significant impact on appetite and nutrition directly or indirectly through adverse effects of certain medications. In addition, one cannot overestimate the terrible effects that bad teeth and inadequate dental care can have on the elderly. Some people cannot and will not eat because of dental pain.

On top of all these issues, aging may also be accompanied by a decreased ability to taste and smell food. There are patients with no apparent socioeconomic barriers or significant medical, surgical, or psychiatric illnesses to explain a decreased appetite, yet they continue to deteriorate in their ability to eat. While the causes for this are not entirely clear, abnormal taste and smell certainly contribute to decreased food intake.

In most situations, deterioration of taste and smell alone does not lead to a state of "cachexia," in which there is wasting of the flesh. Changes in sensory function are usually gradual, sometimes subtle, but almost always contribute to the vulnerability of the elderly to malnutrition. Furthermore, deterioration in taste perception may affect sweet and salty sensations earlier and more severely than other taste sensations. This means that some foods may taste sour and bitter, again resulting in decreased caloric intake.

How Medical Conditions Affect Nutrition in the Elderly

As mentioned earlier, aging is associated with a decline in muscle mass and deterioration in taste, smell, and other sensory functions. These changes are gradual and sometimes subtle. Most of the noticeable changes in nutrition in the elderly occur after a severe illness or with a chronic illness. In fact, chronic illnesses occur more frequently in the elderly population, which is discussed in more depth in chapter 4.10.

Most illnesses in the elderly affect appetite, nutrient absorption, and overall metabolism. Diseases may directly affect the digestive system or indirectly decrease food intake due to fatigue, loss of coordination of body functions, restriction of mobility, pain, nausea, or simply lack of appetite. Conditions that are more frequently encountered in the elderly, such as stroke (interruption of blood flow to the brain causing loss of brain function), heart disease, pneumonia (infection in the lungs), arthritis (painful inflammation of the joints), dementia (decreased ability to think normally), depression, or cancer, may all affect eating behavior.

The elderly are more prone to diseases of the digestive system. Changes in the oral cavity are sometimes of particular concern. Dry mouth, inadequate oral hygiene, poor dental care or poorly fitting dentures, and inflammation of the gums ("gingivitis") can all lead to difficulties with eating, chewing, or swallowing.

Another frequently encountered condition that affects food intake and food absorption in the elderly is a condition called "atrophic gastritis." This condition is found in 20 to 50 percent of people aged sixty-five and above, a rather high percentage. This condition is associated with decreased acid secretion in the stomach, which affects digestion and impairs absorption of some important vitamins and minerals, particularly vitamin B12. Lack of an adequately acidic environment in the intestine may also lead to a condition called bacterial overgrowth. As a result, the absorption of calcium, iron, vitamin B6, and folic acid can be greatly reduced. In addition, the elderly patient with bacterial overgrowth can experience cramping and abdominal pain that further limits food intake. This condition must be treated.

People with metabolic disorders, such as obesity, dyslipidemia, or type 2 diabetes, face an especially daunting challenge in meeting their nutritional needs. The key to meeting this challenge is to balance the need for restricting caloric intake and the need for getting adequate amounts of other essential nutrients from the diet. It is not uncommon to see people who display signs or symptoms of both overnutrition (calories) and undernutrition (vitamins and minerals).

On one hand, people who have had one or more of the metabolic disorders mentioned above would particularly want to avoid caloric overnutrition. Extra calories may exacerbate the existing metabolic problems, possibly leading to serious medical complications such as coronary heart disease, stroke, kidney failure, diabetic eye disease, or foot ulceration and infection. Thus, the health risk of consuming more calories than the body needs is too high to ignore under these particular conditions.

On the other hand, the elderly are more vulnerable than younger persons to vitamin and mineral undernutrition. In addition, whenever there are special constraints on the amount of fat, cholesterol, starch, and/or sugar recommended in the diet, food choices become more limited and meals may not taste as good. Therefore, people who must restrict caloric intake, but are unsure of how to balance their nutritional needs, should consult a physician or a registered dietitian who understands these medical conditions, especially taking into account various cultural and economical conditions.

Polypharmacy and Food-drug Interactions

The term *polypharmacy* refers to the use of multiple medications prescribed by doctors to treat a patient's medical, surgical, or psychiatric illnesses. Usually, it refers to five or more drugs taken by a patient at any given time. On average, elderly Americans age sixty-five and above take two to six prescription drugs plus several over-the-counter medicines on a regular basis.

Polypharmacy is a big concern in nutritional practice for at least two reasons. First, many drugs have unintended adverse effects on appetite. Numerous drugs can cause dry mouth and alter taste function, resulting in poor perception of otherwise palatable foods. Some side effects of medications, such as diarrhea, nausea, and abdominal discomfort, are directly linked to poor food intake and/or absorption. Second, the usual side effects of drugs and drug-drug interactions may be amplified in elderly people due to age-related decline in drug metabolism and excretion. Additionally, drug-nutrient interactions may affect the absorption and metabolism of both the drugs and nutrients. Due to polypharmacy, suboptimal intake and absorption or even frank deficiency of specific nutrients can occur, especially if polypharmacy treatments are chronic.

Physicians treating geriatric patients should make every effort to reduce the number of unnecessary medications for their patients. This practice is important not only for achieving better compliance and adherence to the treatment regimens, but also for better nutritional care of the patients. Even if the prescribed drugs do not directly affect appetite, they may still be a cause of undernutrition, as they may affect other parts of the digestive system. In this regard, physicians should make sure that their patients are not opting for decreasing food intake as an avoidance strategy just because they have abdominal discomfort, nausea, diarrhea, or constipation associated with their medications. Chronic laxative use in the elderly is another cause for tremendous concern. The direct consequence is the impairment of nutrient absorption and increased water and electrolyte loss.

Special Issues with Nursing Home Residents and Long-term Care Patients

Nutritional care and practice for patients in long-term care facilities and nursing home residents deserves a separate discussion. Everything that has been discussed above for the elderly in general also applies to the institutionalized elderly. Challenges for this population are related to their poorer health conditions and impaired activities of daily living. Institutionalized elderly are usually functionally disabled and need assistance in daily living. Nursing homes and long-term care facilities provide daily living care and meal assistance for these seniors. Therefore, nutritional care of these patients is largely delegated to the institutions. Surveys show that undernutrition occurs in significantly higher rates in the institutionalized elderly than in those living independently in the community. This is a serious problem.

Undoubtedly, institutionalized senior citizens are frailer than the free-living elderly, and providing proper nutritional care for them is difficult. Many institutionalized seniors suffer from debilitating physical and/or mental illness. Confusion, depression, and urinary and fecal incontinence are frequently encountered in nursing home residents. All the risk factors for malnutrition discussed in previous sections, such as oral and dental diseases, anorexia, wasting, and polypharmacy, are usually accentuated in this group.

Surveys and studies also show that a lack of understanding of the importance of nutritional care and poor nutritional practices on the part of the managers and staffs of the nursing homes are among the major obstacles toward better care for the institutionalized elderly. The pressure of time felt by the nursing staff due to understaffing often leads to the precedence of any other medical and nursing activity over mealtime assistance. Some institutions delegate the food service completely to the ancillary personnel, depriving the regular nursing staff of the knowledge of how much and what their patients have actually eaten for each meal. In many cases, there are no records of actual food intake, while large portions of food are often left untouched by the patients by the time the mealtime is over.

The solution to the above problem relies both on the willingness of the institutions to make nutritional care a high priority and on the full implementation of the policy. Policies that encourage social interactions during mealtimes, ensure high quality and palatability of the foods, and mandate documenting food consumption have been highly recommended for improving dietary intake in these frail seniors and enhancing their social well-being. Eating is a social activity. The elderly will benefit from eating at a dining table together with others.

If patients are unable to sit at the dining table, trained personnel should accompany the patients at their bedsides during the mealtime instead of having these patients eating alone in silence. The trained personnel should follow appropriate guidelines but also be flexible with their techniques. Some elderly patients may want to maintain some independence and not have full assistance at mealtimes. In these situations, some patience and encouragement from the nursing staff may be just as productive. Helping move the food tray a little closer, opening a can, or helping with anything the individual is physically unable to do may be all that is needed. Some people may simply need encouragement to help them to finish the food in the tray. The job is challenging, but if the institutions make nutritional care a high priority, significant improvements can be made.

General Considerations and Recommendations

As mentioned, the "elderly" are a heterogeneous group. In this group, even for people of the same age, nutritional needs for one can be very different from those for another because of the potential differences in their health and aging status. Therefore, there is no one-size-fits-all nutritional plan. Additionally, a good nutritional plan should take into consideration an individual's cultural and ethnic background, socioeconomic conditions, and family environment. A good plan must not only make nutritional sense but also be sustainable so that it can support the individual's long-term health.

Suggested Readings

AACE Power of Prevention. "Nutrition." http://pop.aace.com/nutrition.php (accessed on October 29, 2008).

Center for Nutrition Policy and Promotion, US Department of Agriculture. "Dietary Guidelines for Americans 2005." www.healthierus.gov/dietaryguidelines (accessed on October 18, 2008).

Nutrition.gov. "Life Stages, Seniors." http://www.nutrition.gov/nal_display/index.php?info_center=11&tax_level=2&tax_subject=395&topic_id=1785&placement_default=0 (accessed on November 2, 2008).

US Department of Agriculture. "My Pyramid Steps to a Healthier You." http://mypyramid.gov (accessed on October 29, 2008).

US Department of Agriculture. "Professional Development Tools. Older Adults." http://snap.nal.usda.gov/nal_display/index.php?info_center=15&tax_level=3&tax_subject=275&topic_id=1336&level3_id=5216 (accessed on November 2, 2008).

Chapter 4.1

Nutrition and Diabetes

Elise M. Brett, MD, FACE, CNSP

Diabetes is a disease in which glucose, a type of sugar in the blood, is not processed normally by the body. Instead, high levels of glucose remain in the bloodstream, and over time, this can cause damage to the eyes, kidneys, nerves, and blood vessels. People with diabetes have a particularly high incidence of heart disease, which is the leading cause of death. Good control of blood glucose with lifestyle modification and/or medication markedly reduces the risk of complications of diabetes. Nutritional management is one of the keys to controlling this disease.

In type 1 diabetes, the body is completely deficient of insulin, the hormone that normally allows glucose to enter the cells. People with type 1 diabetes must take insulin every day or risk a serious illness called diabetic ketoacidosis and ultimately death. In non-diabetics, insulin is normally secreted at steady low levels when one is fasting and then a spike of insulin is produced at mealtimes when carbohydrate is ingested. People with type 1 diabetes obtain the best glucose control when the steady low levels are mimicked with either one or two daily injections of a long-acting insulin or insulin infused continuously via a pump; then, a rapid-acting insulin is taken at mealtimes or given as a bolus with the pump. The mealtime insulin produces a spike that matches the entrance of glucose into the bloodstream as the meal is ingested, and prevents the blood sugar from going up too much after the meal.

Insulin is necessary for the body to process all types of ingested carbohydrate, not just sugars. Carbohydrate-containing foods include starches and sugars. Starches are foods such as bread, rice, and pasta, as well as starchy vegetables such as peas, corn, and beans. Sugars include sweets like candy, cookies, and cakes, as well as natural sugars such as those contained in fruits and fruit juices.

"Carbohydrate counting" is one method used by people with type 1 diabetes to match the insulin dose correctly to the amount of carbohydrate ingested. Carbohydrates that are eaten are counted in grams, and the dose is calculated using an "insulin to carbohydrate ratio." This is trickier than it may seem because portion sizes can be difficult to estimate (especially in restaurants), there are often hidden carbohydrates in prepared meals, and the other components of the meal (fat, protein, and fiber) may alter the absorption rate of the carbohydrates. Nevertheless, by using this method, people with type 1 diabetes can essentially eat what they want, when they want, and still obtain good glucose control.

In type 2 diabetes, there are several defects that alter the uptake of glucose. Although the body produces insulin, there is a relative insulin deficiency, which tends to progress over time. There is insulin resistance in the muscle and fat tissues, meaning these tissues do not take up glucose normally. There is also insulin resistance in the liver, which causes it to release too much glucose into the bloodstream. Lastly, there are special gut hormones, that normally slow the absorption of glucose and inhibit appetite, and this effect may be impaired in type 2 diabetes. Most people who have type 2 diabetes are overweight or obese, and the excess body fat tends to worsen the insulin resistance. In many patients, weight loss improves glucose control. Weight loss, along with regular exercise, can also prevent or delay the onset of diabetes.

The type of diet to best manage type 2 diabetes depends on the person's body weight and the type of medication regimen being used to treat the diabetes. Early in the course of the disease, most people with type 2 diabetes can be treated with oral medication. There are now medications available to target each of the different defects that cause the disease. In general, people with type 2 diabetes treated with oral agents are best managed nutritionally by eating well-balanced meals spaced throughout the day so as to not overload carbohydrates at any one time and cause a spike in blood sugar. Most people with type 2 diabetes must also restrict calories to lose weight or avoid excess weight gain. People who take a sulfonylurea-type medication, which continuously stimulates insulin secretion, must not skip meals or they could develop a dangerously low blood sugar. Those who use other oral medications can usually skip meals without any adverse effect.

Many people with type 2 diabetes will eventually require insulin treatment as the disease progresses. Some people with type 2 diabetes will be treated with a basal-bolus regimen similar to that of type 1 diabetes, in which case dietary management is similar. Others will be treated with one or two injections per day of an intermediate acting insulin, which has a peak action around four to six hours after injection. If treated with an intermediate acting insulin or a premixed insulin (such as 70/30 insulin or 75/25 insulin) in the morning, it is essential that the person not skip meals or there is a risk of low blood glucose. Similarly, if an intermediate acting insulin is taken at dinner or bedtime, a bedtime snack is often required to prevent low glucose during the night. With other treatment regimens, a bedtime snack is not usually needed.

Since people with diabetes are at higher risk for heart disease, it is also necessary to be cautious with fat intake. Saturated fats, those contained in animal products and dairy products, raise cholesterol and contribute to heart disease but are contained in the protein sources of most people's diets. In general, it is better to more often choose lower fat sources such as fish or poultry without the skin instead of red meat, to choose fat-free milk or low-fat cottage cheese or yogurts instead of hard cheeses, and to choose egg whites as opposed to whole eggs. However, it is not necessary to completely avoid any particular foods but just limit intake.

Monounsaturated fatty acids, such as those found in nuts, avocados, or olive oils, actually lower cholesterol and are a healthy replacement for some dietary carbohydrate. When possible, olive oil or canola oil should be substituted for butter in cooking. Trans fats, such as those found in margarines and other hydrogenated oils, are the most unhealthy types of fat, and their intake should be severely limited.

Fiber is a component of carbohydrate that is particularly beneficial for people with diabetes because it tends to slow the absorption of carbohydrate and even out the level of blood sugar. Fiber also helps to maintain a healthy gastrointestinal tract. Most people do not get enough fiber in the diet. About 30 grams per day is recommended. Reading Nutrition Facts labels on store-bought foods will tell you how much fiber is in the food (see chapter 1.2, "Reading a Nutrition Facts Label"). Fiber-containing foods include fruits with the skins, whole-grain breads, cereals, vegetables, and beans.

In summary, there is no one "diabetic diet." There are no foods that need to be completely restricted for people with diabetes. Products labeled as "sugar-free" or "diabetic" may still contain large amounts of carbohydrate and are not necessarily better for the diet. The key for most people is to keep intake of higher saturated fat foods and high carbohydrate foods in moderation and to focus on eating well-balanced meals and losing weight, if needed. Although gram for gram the effect on blood glucose is the same for all carbohydrates, better carbohydrate choices include fruits, vegetables, and whole-grain products because these foods also contain vitamins and fiber.

For people with type 2 diabetes who are overweight, even a 5 to 10 percent loss of body weight will often substantially improve glucose control. This can generally be achieved by reducing overall caloric intake by 500 calories per day to induce weight loss of one to two pounds per week. Reading food labels or using a reference book can usually help one make better food choices and lose weight.

Suggested Readings

Goedt FT, Polin BS. *The Joslin Diabetes Quick and Easy Cookbook.* Simon & Schuster, New York, 1998.

Holler HJ, Pastors JG. Diabetes Medical Nutrition Therapy. American Dietetic Association, 1997.

Mechanick JI, Brett EM. *Nutritional Strategies for the Diabetic & Prediabetic Patient.* CRC Taylor & Francis, New York, 2006.

Poirier LM, Coburn KM. Women & Diabetes. American Diabetes Association, Alexandria, VA, 2000.

Power of Prevention, Endocrine Health: Diabetes. http://www.powerofprevention.com/diabetes.php (accessed on September 2, 2008).

Warshaw HS, Webb R. The Diabetes Food & Nutrition Bible. American Diabetes Association, Alexandria, VA, 2001.

Chapter 4.2

Nutrition and Obesity

Maria L. Collazo-Clavell, MD

A healthy weight is determined by using a calculation called "body mass index," or "BMI" for short. This calculation takes an individual's height and weight into consideration, and is computed the following way (may also refer to http://www.nhlbi.nih.gov/guidelines/obesity/bmi_tbl.htm for a table of BMI values or the AACE Web site http://www.powerofprevention.com/bmi.php for a "BMI calculator"):

1. Divide your weight in pounds by 2.2 to get your weight in kilograms (example: 150 pounds equals 68.2 kilograms).
2. Calculate the number of total inches in your height—there are 12 inches for every foot and then add the rest of the inches (example: 5 feet 6 inches equals 66 inches total).
3. Multiply your total inches of height by 2.54 to get the total number of centimeters of height (example: 66 inches times 2.54 equals 167.6 centimeters).
4. Divide the number of centimeters of height by 100 to get the number of meters of height (example: 167.6 centimeters divided by 100 equals 1.676 meters).
5. Multiply the number of meters of height by itself (square it) to get "meters-squared" for "height-squared" (example: 1.676 times 1.676 equals 2.81).
6. Finally, divide the weight in kilograms by the height-squared as meters-squared to get the final BMI (example: 68.2 kilograms divided by 2.81 equals 24.4).
7. The mathematical equation looks like this: BMI = Weight (kg)/Height-Squared (M^2).
8. The interpretation of the result is:

   a. underweight is a BMI of less than 18.5
   b. normal weight is a BMI of 18.5 to 24.9
   c. overweight is a BMI of 25 to 29.9, and
   d. obese is a BMI of 30 and over.

People with BMI values of 30 or greater are obese and are at risk for developing health problems like diabetes, high blood pressure, high cholesterol, and even some types of cancer. Obesity also increases the chances of developing heart disease and dying early. The most dangerous type of obesity is "central obesity" or "apple shape." This type of excess fat is associated with insulin resistance and the "metabolic syndrome." The metabolic syndrome is a group of risk factors for coronary artery disease including large waist, elevated blood triglycerides, low HDL-cholesterol, elevated blood glucose (but not necessarily diabetes), and high blood pressure. Several different specific definitions of metabolic syndrome have been published.

The number of Americans who are above a healthy weight continues to rise. When last reported, more than six out of ten adult Americans were either overweight or obese. The same is true for children and adolescents. Many factors have contributed to the United States becoming a heavier nation. The two main factors are changes in eating habits and changes in physical activity.

Over the past twenty years, several changes in eating habits have led to weight gain. Today, people are eating larger amounts of food, food that is higher in calories and food that is often prepared outside of the home. People are also drinking large amounts of calories in sweetened beverages, such as soda pop and juices, which are replacing water or more nutritious beverages, like milk.

Society is less physically active. Children, adolescents, and adults do not participate in as much physical activity during their free time, such as structured exercise or neighborhood games, as in the past. Schools have decreased the requirements for physical education classes. Instead, free time is spent engaging in sedentary activities like TV watching, playing video games, or working on a computer. Jobs have also become less physically demanding. Simply put, eating larger amounts of food, high in calories and with less opportunity to burn off those extra calories, have led to the increasing number of people who are overweight or obese.

Nutrition and Overall Health

The goal of healthy eating, even in people with a normal BMI, is to provide our bodies with the energy and nutrients needed to function properly and protect against disease. In 2005, the United States Department of Agriculture released the new Dietary Guidelines for Americans emphasizing foods that promote good health. These guidelines encouraged the intake of fruits, vegetables, whole grains, fat-free or low-fat milk products, lean meats, fish, nuts, and legumes (like beans), while limiting the intake of foods high in salt, cholesterol, saturated fats, and *trans* fats. Sticking with such a diet can help control weight; lower an elevated blood pressure, blood sugar, or cholesterol; and lower the chance of having a heart attack and some types of cancer. Although most Americans are aware of the diet they should follow, most find it difficult to do so.

Nutrition for Weight Management

The majority of Americans have attempted to change their eating habits in the hopes of losing weight several times throughout their lives. For most, their initial efforts at dietary change are successful at achieving weight loss but cannot be sustained. This leads to weight regain and frustration. Success at weight management requires a long-term commitment to the dietary changes instituted as well as gradual increases in physical activity.

No one diet works for everyone. Truth be known, all diets work while followed since they are associated with less calories being consumed. However, *dietary changes should not only promote weight loss but also promote good health!* So, the goal should be gradual changes toward the current recommended intakes for fruits, vegetables, low-fat dairy products, and lean meats, while controlling calories from foods with low nutritional value, such as sweetened beverages, alcohol, and high-fat foods.

Where to Start

Keeping a diary or journal of current eating habits and learning about their calorie and fat content can allow a person to identify areas for potential change. A person can identify the calorie and fat content of foods by reading food labels and searching for nutrition information of foods served at local restaurants or at their corresponding Web sites. There are also several Web sites where you can find the nutrition information of common and uncommonly prepared foods (see Suggested Readings below). Although it requires effort, several studies have confirmed that keeping a diet record is associated with greater success at weight loss.

How Can a Person Identify What Changes to Make?

Dietary change to achieve weight loss requires cutting back calories. Generally, it is recommended to cut back by at least 250 to 500 calories per day. If this is done consistently, this amount of calorie restriction can lead to an average weight loss of half a pound to a full pound per week.

For some, greater calorie restriction will be possible if many areas are identified for relatively easy calorie restriction. For example, an individual who drinks two to three bottles of a 20-ounce regular soda can cut back over 500 calories a day by switching to a diet soda alone. For others, it may be more challenging to find ways to cut back 250 to 500 calories a day.

It is important to remember that dietary and physical activity changes instituted need to be maintained over the long term in order to maintain a healthy weight. So, tackling gradual changes over time is best. In general, losing between half a pound and up to even two pounds per week is considered safe.

Portion Control

Portion control limits the intake of routinely consumed foods. This is a straightforward way of cutting back calories. Knowing the recommended serving sizes of foods can serve as a realistic goal for healthy eating. However, *any* change that reduces calories and improves the amount of health-promoting foods is beneficial. Portion control is particularly important for starchy foods such as pasta, rice, potatoes, and bread. These foods are often over consumed and are staples in meals, allowing many opportunities for change. Meat servings present another opportunity for change.

Portion control may not be as easy as it sounds. How can a person control portions that are served at a local restaurant? How can portion sizes be controlled at home? How does a person order a half portion at the restaurant, share a meal, or eat half of a meal and take the other half home? Can a person get into the habit of preparing less food at home? Recognizing and planning for situations that may promote overeating will help achieve the goals discussed. Ultimately, changing unhealthy behaviors that have become routine is the key to success.

Food Selection and Introduction of Healthier Alternatives

As you start keeping a diet record, it will become clear which foods tend to be high in calories and should be limited and which foods you may not be getting enough of and need to increase. Foods that are high in fat will be higher in calories. Gradually switching to lower fat alternatives is another way of cutting back calories. But, do not be misled by food labels since not all low-fat foods are low in calories. Completely giving up a food that is enjoyed may not lead to long-term success. It is more productive to limit the amount of a food that is enjoyed or how often this food is eaten as you try to find other options that satisfy you and still allow you to stick with dietary goals.

Most Americans do not eat enough fruits and vegetables on a daily basis. Several obstacles are often noted, including the perception that fresh produce is expensive and can easily spoil. Introducing fruits into a routine day may actually prove to be one of the easiest changes one can make. Fruits generally do not require preparation and can be easily taken to work or school. The key is to get into the habit of purchasing fruits and have them easily available for an entire family. Examples are the classic fruit bowl on the dinner table. Buying fruits that are in season can save money and will naturally introduce some variety as the seasons change. Introduce fruits as part of a usual meal as a side dish, dessert, or as an afternoon snack. Developing a taste for fruits may be harder on some individuals. It is okay to improve the taste of fruits by adding an artificial sweetener or a small amount of sugar, but do not lose track of your goals.

Many of the same ideas can work toward increasing the intake of vegetables. Learn the appropriate portion sizes for vegetables and introduce them gradually. The nice thing about non-starchy vegetables is that they can be consumed as desired with very few calories. Vegetables such as carrots, broccoli, and cauliflower, raw or steamed, can be served with a lower calorie dressing on the side or eaten alone as a snack. Salad greens are also an easy alternative, but beware of all the "extras." High-calorie and high-fat dressings, cheese, and nuts add to the calorie value of a meal and can prevent people from achieving their eating goals. Finding ways to introduce other vegetables, such as asparagus, green peppers, and red peppers, to meals can take some time, but when the opportunity presents itself, like with a new recipe or social event, try them.

Food Preparation

Introducing new recipes and healthier ways to prepare meals requires the most effort and is often one of the last things to do. However, this strategy will add variety to meals and expand eating options. After all the dietary restrictions people are advised to consider, introducing new foods, indeed healthy foods, should be a welcome change. Easy targets include limiting frying and opting for baking, broiling, and grilling. Replace the use of butter in food preparation with healthier oils, like olive, canola, or sunflower oil. Try seasonings other than salt to add flavor to meals. Look for recipes in the newspaper, in magazines, or on Web sites. If there is a particular cuisine that is enjoyed, then invest in a recipe book. There is no need to overdo this at the beginning, and pacing these changes is important. Select recipes that are easy to shop for, prepare, and have a high likelihood to be welcomed by family. Be prepared for a lot of trial and error. Do not be discouraged if a recipe does not work out.

Registered Dietitian

Changing eating habits can be overwhelming. If this is too much to handle, especially in the presence of other life-stresses related to work or at home, then recruiting the help of a dietitian should be considered. A registered dietitian can help a person start a plan and provide ongoing support. Rarely is one visit with a registered dietitian enough. In fact, studies looking at weight management include visits with a registered dietitian at least every other month. Do not be afraid to use this valuable resource and go prepared with specific questions regarding changes you want to make.

Obstacles to Change

Most individuals know what they should do to improve their eating habits. So, why don't they? The answer lies in obstacles. Making changes takes effort, especially when there is nothing to make things easier. The current environment is not particularly supportive of healthy eating initiatives. Busy lives, as well as home and work responsibilities, can easily sabotage all the good intentions an individual may have. People should try to recognize their own individual obstacles that pose a threat to success. Make a commitment to change, think through the obstacles, and come up with potential solutions. Obstacles should not ultimately discourage changes that lead to healthy eating; they just need to be identified and then tackled.

An initial weight loss goal should be 5 to 10 percent of the initial body weight. As an example, for a weight of two hundred pounds, 5 percent weight loss is ten pounds, and 10 percent weight loss is twenty pounds. This is definitely a realistic goal. This amount of weight loss has been shown to improve many aspects of health including preventing type 2 diabetes. However, disappointment with this amount of weight loss despite the hard work at changing eating habits can be discouraging. It is strongly recommended to tackle the first ten pounds of weight loss before thinking about the last ten pounds of weight loss. Plateaus in weight loss will happen, and it is important not to feel defeated by them.

Some obstacles cannot be tackled without help. Family and friends can help. Healthy eating can be a family affair, which can reward positive changes in spouses and children. One can choose different activities or different restaurants at which to socialize with friends. Obviously, doctors can help their patients stick with positive lifestyle changes by providing a referral to a registered dietitian, reviewing medications since some may promote weight gain and others can be started to help lose weight, and simply talking about proven motivational strategies for weight loss.

Measuring Success

Although weight loss is the motivation, people should not measure their success by the number on the scale. This can be discouraging. Rather, people should look at the changes made in eating and physical activity habits. People should take pride when their children, start eating more fruits and vegetables and recognizing what healthy eating really means. Physical activity should be increased, and there is also great pride taken in this lifestyle change. This reduces the risk for diabetes, heart disease, and even dying early. A word of caution: people should not set themselves up for failure. Realistic goals should be set and strategies started at a gradual pace.

Conclusion

Although challenging, improving eating and activity habits can have a profound impact on health and well-being today and into the future. People should be armed with reliable information, be surrounded with support, and stay motivated to make each day a better one.

Suggested Readings

About.com. "Weight Loss." http://weightloss.about.com/od/eatsmart/a/blcalintake_2.htm (accessed on September 1, 2008).

Calorie King. www.calorieking.com (accessed on September 1, 2008).

Center for Nutrition Policy and Promotion, US Department of Agriculture. "Dietary Guidelines for Americans 2005." www.healthierus.gov/dietaryguidelines (accessed on October 18, 2008).

Eisenson HJ, Binks M. *The Duke Diet*. Ballantine Books, New York, 2007.

Kushner RF, Kushner N, Blatner DJ. Counseling overweight adults: The lifestyle patterns approach and toolkit. American Dietetic Association, September 2008.

Power of Prevention, Endocrine Health: Obesity. http://www.powerofprevention.com/obesity.php (accessed on September 2, 2008).

The Obesity Society. http://www.obesity.org/ (accessed on September 2, 2008).

Chapter 4.3

Nutrition and Hypertension

Osama Hamdy, MD, PhD, FACE

Hypertension is the term used to refer to high blood pressure (BP). About 72 million US adults suffer from hypertension (approximately one in every four individuals). Table 1 shows the current definition of normal blood pressure, pre-hypertension (a condition that does not require pharmacological therapy but may eventually lead to hypertension), and hypertension.

A Few Facts about Hypertension

- Blood pressure usually increases with age. About 75 percent of all US adults have hypertension by age seventy or older.
- Hypertension is more prevalent, more severe, and diagnosed at a younger age among African Americans than Caucasians.
- Due to the usual lack of symptoms, one in every three people with hypertension does not know that her/his blood pressure is high.
- Untreated hypertension leads to devastating complications like stroke, heart attack, heart failure, and kidney failure.
- At least 1 million persons die every year in relation to hypertension or its complications.
- Only 27 percent of hypertensive patients have their BP under good control.
- Ninety-five percent of hypertension is called primary ("essential") hypertension, which means we do not know what causes it. However, inheritance and poor lifestyle may contribute to the hypertensive state.
- Secondary hypertension refers to high blood pressure caused by other conditions or medications. Examples include sleep apnea, hyperactive or hypoactive thyroid, abnormal constriction of the aorta, some kidney diseases, hormone-producing tumors of the adrenal gland, pre-eclampsia and eclampsia (high BP in pregnancy), chronic use of some over-the-counter medications, oral steroids, and oral contraceptive pills. Secondary hypertension accounts for 5 percent of all hypertension cases.

What Are the Basic Principles of Nutrition and Hypertension?

Proper nutrition and healthy lifestyle play major roles in lowering blood pressure in hypertensive patients and in preventing hypertension in pre-hypertensive individuals. Table 2 shows the basic principles of nutrition and lifestyle changes and their potential effect on blood pressure.

What Is the DASH Diet Plan?

DASH refers to Dietary Approaches to Stop Hypertension. The DASH eating plan is a diet rich in fruits, vegetables (8–10 servings per day), and low-fat or non-fat dairy products with a reduced content of dietary cholesterol as well as saturated fat (less than 10 percent of caloric intake) and total fat (about 27 percent of caloric intake). It is rich in potassium, calcium, and magnesium. The diet also includes whole gains, nuts, fish, poultry, and a small amount of red meat. The total salt in the DASH diet is 7.5 grams, and the total calories per day are around 2,000. The DASH eating plan has BP-reducing effects similar to treatment with a single medicine. The systolic and diastolic BP in hypertensive individuals who participated in the DASH study were reduced by 11.4 and 5.5 mmHg, respectively. In individuals with borderline high blood pressure, the systolic BP decreased by 3.5 mmHg and their diastolic BP decreased by 2 mmHg.

Other Considerations in Dietary Intervention

Dietary Potassium

Increased dietary potassium has shown to be beneficial in people with hypertension, as long as kidney function is normal. The amount of potassium used in the DASH diet was 2.5 times higher than in the ordinary diet in the US. Foods that are rich in potassium include bananas, oranges, apricots, avocado, kiwi, artichokes, beets, figs, pears, spinach, prunes, potatoes, orange juice, milk, and plain yogurt.

Licorice

Natural licorice raises blood pressure, sometimes significantly. It contains the chemical "glycyrrhizin," which causes the body to retain sodium (and therefore fluids) and to lose potassium. People with hypertension, particularly those taking diuretics (water pills), would probably be far more susceptible to such effects and should, therefore, avoid candy, beverages, and smokeless tobacco that contain natural licorice. Domestically produced licorice candy is generally made with artificial flavor and does *not* contain natural licorice.

Tyramine-containing Food

Tyramine-containing foods may cause a rise in blood pressure. That rise could be more severe in people treated with a group of compounds used for treatment of depression called MAOI (monoamine oxidase inhibitors). Tyramine-containing foods include hard or aged cheese; cheddar cheese; aged or cured meats (e.g., air-dried sausage); aged, pickled, or smoked meats (e.g., salami); broad (fava) bean pods; marmite concentrated yeast extract; sauerkraut; soy sauce and soy bean products; vermouth; beer (dark more than light, on tap more than in bottles because tyramine is adsorbed to glass); and red wine more than white wine.

Mediterranean Diet

The Mediterranean eating style significantly reduces the risk of further heart disease in individuals who have already had a heart attack. The Mediterranean diet was also found to reduce bad cholesterol (LDL-cholesterol) and has some positive impact on BP. This effect is as much as with the DASH diet, although these diets have never been directly compared in a scientific study. The Mediterranean diet is similar to the American Heart Association's Step I diet, but it contains less cholesterol and has monounsaturated fatty acids (MUFAs) and polyunsaturated fatty acids (PUFAs) like linolenic acid, which is also an omega-3 fatty acid. Fat sources for MUFAs include olive oil, canola oil, and certain nuts, particularly walnuts.

The key components of the Mediterranean diet include:

- eating a generous amount of fruits and vegetables,
- consuming healthy fats such as olive oil and canola oil,
- eating small portions of nuts,
- drinking red wine in moderation,
- consuming very little red meat, and
- eating fish on a regular basis.

A Prudent Diet for Hypertension

Prudent eating is characterized by a higher intake of cruciferous vegetables (broccoli, brussels sprouts, cabbage, and cauliflower, for example), greens, carrots, and fresh fruits and a lower intake of meat (red meat), meat products, sweets, high-fat dairy, and white bread (white bread and unrefined cereal). Most of the protein sources in a prudent dietary pattern are from lean red meat or fish and skinless poultry. This dietary pattern has been proven to be much better in reducing hypertension and cardiovascular risk than a Western dietary pattern, characterized by processed and red meats, eggs, potatoes, and refined grains.

Suggested Readings

Cleveland Clinic. "High Blood Pressure and Nutrition." http://my.clevelandclinic.org/disorders/Hypertension_High_Blood_Pressure/hic_High_Blood_Pressure_and_Nutrition.aspx (accessed on September 21, 2008).

MedlinePlus. "High Blood Pressure." http://www.nlm.nih.gov/medlineplus/highbloodpressure.html (accessed on September 21, 2008).

The DASH Diet Eating Plan. http://dashdiet.org/ (accessed on September 21, 2008).

Your Guide to Lowering High Blood Pressure. http://www.nhlbi.nih.gov/hbp/prevent/sodium/sodium.htm (accessed on September 21, 2008).

Table 1. How high is high for blood pressure?

	"Top Number" Systolic BP (mmHg)	"Bottom Number" Diastolic BP (mmHg)
Normal	**< 120**	**< 80**
Pre-Hypertension	**120-139**	**80-89**
Hypertension	**≥ 140**	**≥ 90**

Table 2. Effects of lifestyle on high blood pressure.

Nutrition and lifestyle modifications	Target	Expected reduction in BP
Dietary sodium reduction	Reduce dietary sodium intake to no more than 2.4 gm of sodium or 6 gm of sodium chloride (salt).	4–9 mmHg
DASH eating plan	Eat a diet rich in fruits and vegetables, and low in fat dairy products with a reduced content of saturated and total fat	8–14 mmHg
Weight reduction	Achieve normal body weight; a body mass index (18.5–24.9 kg/m2). However, weight loss of as little as 4.5 kg (10 lbs) reduces BP and/or prevents hypertension in a large proportion of overweight persons	5–20 mmHg/10 kg (22 lbs)
Physical activity	Engage in regular moderate intensity physical activity such as brisk walking at rate of 3 miles/hour (at least 30-45 min per day in most days of the week with a total of >150 minutes/week)	2–8 mmHg
Moderation of alcohol consumption	Limit alcohol consumption to <1 oz (30 mL) of ethanol /day or approximately 2 drinks (e.g., 24 oz beer, 10 oz wine, or 3 oz 80-proof liquor) per day in most men, and to no more than 1 drink (e.g., 12 oz of beer, 5 oz of wine, and 1.5 oz of 80-proof liquor) per day in women and lighter weight persons.	2–4 mmHg
Stop smoking		Reduces complications of hypertension

Chapter 4.4

Nutrition and Kidney Disease

Jeffrey I. Mechanick, MD, FACP, FACE, FACN
Elise M. Brett, MD, FACE, CNSP

The kidneys are vital organs in the body that are mainly responsible for the elimination of waste products that circulate directly in the bloodstream. Specialized structures in the kidney called "nephrons" perform the basic functions. First, blood is "filtered" in the "glomerulus" of the nephron, and this produces a "filtrate" solution. This filtrate solution then moves through specialized tubes in the nephron, called "tubules." These tubules can bring certain chemicals back from the filtrate ("resorption") into the blood and can also eliminate certain chemicals from the blood back into the filtrate ("secretion"). The net effect of filtration, resorption, and secretion is "excretion" of waste products in the form of "urine." Urine passes out of each nephron's collecting duct into a larger tube called the ureter. The right kidney's ureter and the left kidney's ureter both pass urine into a larger sac called the "bladder." Here, urine collects until the person feels the urge to urinate. Then, urine passes out of the body through a tube called the "urethra."

Several diseases can affect the kidney either directly or indirectly. For instance, there are certain diseases of the glomerulus or the tubules that can lead to kidney failure and are called "renal" diseases. These processes can occur rapidly, as with infections, or more slowly, as with immune disorders, such as "lupus." Sometimes, diseases that affect other parts of the body, such as diabetes or high blood pressure, can also slowly affect kidney function and lead to "chronic kidney disease," or CKD.

There are five different stages of CKD, which are related to increasing severity of the kidney impairment, with the first stage being the mildest and the final fifth stage representing near complete "kidney failure" and the need for "dialysis." There are two basic types of dialysis, in which the blood is artificially filtered: "hemodialysis," where the blood goes directly into a dialysis machine, and "peritoneal dialysis," where the fluid in the abdomen that surrounds the intestines is exchanged slowly with another solution. These "renal replacement therapies" remove waste products in the blood similar to what a kidney can do.

Nutritional factors can influence the rate at which CKD can become harmful to an individual. In addition, CKD can influence what healthy eating is for a given person. The following nutritional principles apply to CKD.

What Is the Correct Amount of Calories to Consume Daily with CKD?

In general, patients with CKD who have not yet required dialysis need to limit protein so there is always a possibility that total calories are also limited in the process. If total calories are limited too much, then the body naturally breaks down muscle tissue and even internal organs in order to create metabolic fuel.

People with advanced CKD, especially those on dialysis, can develop a form of inflammation and malnutrition called "protein-energy wasting." This occurs in up to half of these people and can increase the likelihood of hospitalization or even premature death. Two processes result from the inflammation associated with advanced CKD: increased breakdown of cells and decreased appetite. In fact, doctors sometimes prescribe an appetite stimulant called "megestrol acetate" to help promote weight gain.

Normally, people need about 30 calories per kilogram of dry body weight per day (or 2,300 calories a day for a 175-pound person [175 pounds = 77 kilograms; 77 x 30 = about 2,300]. This is based on "dry" weight and does not include the excess water weight that occurs when swelling is present. If a person is overweight or obese, then the weight used is the ideal body weight, which a doctor or dietitian can calculate based on the body mass index (BMI). People with advanced CKD on dialysis may need more than 30 calories per kilogram of dry body weight.

People with CKD should try to maintain a healthy weight by adjusting their total calories up or down based on actual weight change. A healthy weight is one that is not too lean (above a BMI of 18.5) and not overweight (below a BMI of 25), where BMI is weight in kilograms divided by the height in meters-squared (so a 6-foot person [72 inches x 2.54 centimeters per inch = 183 centimeters = 1.83 meters = 3.35 meters-squared] weighing 180 pounds [180 divided by 2.2 = 82 kilograms] has a normal BMI of 24.5 [82 divided by 3.35]). If someone has trouble consuming adequate calories through regular food, a canned liquid supplement designed for people with kidney disease can be added to the diet and may help promote weight gain.

What Is the Right Amount of Protein?

In general, patients with CKD who are not receiving renal replacement therapy should limit their protein intake since high amounts of protein waste places a burden on kidneys to eliminate protein waste products. The amount of protein a normal person requires is about 1 gram per kilogram body weight, or about 80 grams a day for a 175-pound person. People with early CKD may need to restrict their protein intake to 0.6 to 0.8 grams of protein per kilogram body weight, or about 50 to 60 grams a day for a 175-pound person. Even though dietary protein should be limited, it should not be limited too much or else muscle mass, organ function, and immunity can be harmed. People already on dialysis will need more protein, as high as 1.2 grams per kilogram body weight, or about 95 grams a day for a 175-pound person.

High biological value protein can be found in virtually all animal sources of protein, such as eggs, dairy (milk products and cheese), and meats (beef, lamb, pork, poultry, and fish). High biological value protein can also be found in certain plants, especially beans and bean products, such as tofu (bean curd). However, beans and tofu have higher amounts of potassium, phosphorus, and magnesium in them so intake of these foods may actually need to be limited depending on the severity of CKD. High biological value protein is preferred since it provides all of the essential amino acids, which are the building blocks of protein.

What Other Nutritional Concerns Are There with CKD?

Sodium

Since high blood pressure and dietary sodium, or salt (which is chemically "sodium chloride"), intake are related, people with CKD should limit the amount of sodium in their food. Kidney tubules normally hold on to sodium in a process called "sodium resorption." Therefore, many people with CKD will need to limit their sodium intake. Here are some ways in which to do so:

- Avoid salting food with a saltshaker on the table.
- Check the Nutrition Facts labels on foods; most food seasonings, such as garlic or onion salt, soy or teriyaki sauces, or "steak" sauces, are high in sodium, and most canned foods, dehydrated soups, and some frozen foods are high in sodium.
- Avoid most "junk" foods, "fast" foods, and "snack" foods, as they are typically high in sodium.

People with CKD should not simply use a "salt-substitute" without reading the Nutrition Facts label carefully, since they frequently contain potassium, which must also be limited in some patients with CKD.

What foods are relatively low in sodium? Fresh fruits and vegetables are generally low in sodium, though some have a fair amount of potassium so one may need to be familiar with the nutrient content of these foods and discuss this with a registered dietitian (RD). Fresh herbs and spices, pepper sauce, lemon juice, and other natural flavorings will have less sodium than store-bought sauces and "salts."

Potassium

This electrolyte is essentially a waste product in the body since most of the potassium in the body is found inside the cell, so when cells break down they release all of their potassium into the bloodstream. The kidneys normally function to eliminate potassium in the urine, but with CKD, blood potassium levels can increase too high—this is called "hyperkalemia." High potassium levels are dangerous to the heart and can cause abnormal heartbeats. Therefore, a critical dietary limitation with CKD is to eat foods that are relatively low in potassium. The amount of potassium restriction that is needed ultimately depends on the severity of CKD. Since certain medications can also raise the potassium level, all medications must be reviewed with a doctor. Foods that are high or low in potassium are provided in the table below.

Phosphorus

This electrolyte is also a metabolic waste product, and the kidney eliminates excess phosphorus in order to maintain normal levels in the bloodstream. When there is CKD, blood phosphorus levels become too high, and this can contribute to bone loss and also form harmful complexes with calcium that irritate the skin. Dietary phosphorus can be limited by avoiding foods relatively high in phosphorus:

- Dairy products (not including non-dairy creamers)
- Legumes (beans, peas, and lentils)
- Nuts, including peanut butter
- Beer, cola, and hot chocolate

If the phosphorus levels are too high, a doctor may prescribe medicines that lower phosphorus levels ("phosphate-binders"), but the patient may still need to avoid foods high in phosphorus.

Calcium

People with CKD may develop problems with bone health. Several reasons account for this: increased phosphorus levels, increased levels of parathyroid hormone, and decreased production of activated vitamin D. Foods that are rich in calcium can improve bone health in people with CKD, but since dairy products are also high in phosphorus, the use of calcium supplements is frequently recommended.

Fluids

Generally speaking, fluids do not need to be limited with early stages of CKD. If swelling occurs or CKD becomes more advanced, then fluid requirements should be discussed with a doctor.

Vitamins

If a person's diet is adequate with respect to total calories and protein, and balanced with respect to the various food groups (meats, dairy, grains, fruits, vegetables, and oils), it is very unlikely that he or she will develop a vitamin deficiency and, therefore, will not require a vitamin supplement. However, since people with advanced CKD frequently have limitations imposed on their diet, they may be at increased risk for certain vitamin deficiencies, mainly vitamin D and the B-complex vitamins. Taking vitamins that are not needed can be harmful. For instance, too much vitamin A can be bad for the bones, and too much activated vitamin D can cause abnormally high blood calcium levels. These are issues best discussed with a doctor and not left up to impulsive purchasing of vitamins in the health-food store merely because they claim to be beneficial.

Kidney Stones

Kidney stones are hard masses composed of different substances that are formed in the kidney. The most common types of kidney stones are composed of calcium and oxalate or uric acid. These stones pass from the kidney through the ureter to the bladder and are then excreted through the urethra along with the urine. Passage of a kidney stone is typically associated with excruciating pain. Sometimes stones can cause serious problems if they block the ureter.

Roughly 12 percent of men and 6 percent of women in the US will have a kidney stone in their lifetimes. Certain people, such as those with inflammatory bowel disease, metabolic syndrome, gout, primary hyperparathyroidism, or those who have undergone intestinal resection or bariatric surgery are at particularly high risk for kidney stones. People who have had a kidney stone have approximately a 50 percent chance of having another stone in the next ten years.

The best treatment for kidney stones is prevention. Several modifications of diet can decrease the chance for recurrence of calcium and uric acid stones. Increasing fluid intake is helpful with all types of stone prevention. People who have had kidney stones will benefit from increasing urine volume to 2 to 3 liters per day. To do this, one must drink 3 to 4 liters (approximately 12–16 cups) of water per day. It is especially important to increase fluid intake with meals. Larger meals require greater fluid intake.

Diets high in animal protein also increase the risk for kidney stones by increasing the amount of calcium and uric acid in the urine. Consumption of organ meats particularly increases this risk. People who have had kidney stones should limit protein to no more than 1 gram per kilogram per day (that is not more than 70 grams per day for a 70-kilogram man).

Ideally, meals should be well spaced throughout the day to decrease the chance for stone formation. People who do not eat for most of the day and then consume one large meal in the evening are more likely to get a kidney stone because the urine becomes overloaded with kidney stone-forming substances.

Excess dietary salt causes the kidneys to put extra calcium in the urine, increasing the risk for calcium stones. People who have had calcium kidney stones should reduce their intake of sodium to less than 2 grams per day. Paradoxically, including calcium in the diet decreases the risk for calcium-oxalate kidney stones. This is because calcium intake reduces the amount of oxalate in the urine. However, people who have had calcium kidney stones should avoid overloads of calcium at any one time. Dietary calcium intake of 800 to 1200 milligrams of elemental calcium per day is probably optimal.

Some people who have high levels of oxalate in the urine can reduce their chance of recurrent stones by reducing dietary intake of oxalate or at least keeping high-oxalate foods well spaced throughout the day. High oxalate foods include rhubarb, peanuts, pecans, tea, beets, berries, chocolate, sweet potatoes, spinach, collard greens, and eggplant. Excess supplementation of vitamin C (greater than 1,000 milligrams per day) increases urine oxalate and may increase the risk for calcium oxalate kidney stones. For unclear reasons, consumption of apple juice and grapefruit juice is also associated with a greater chance of kidney stones.

People who have had a kidney stone should have basic blood testing to rule out systemic diseases associated with kidney stones. For people who have had recurrent stones, a complete metabolic evaluation including analysis of the urine is required. Typically, certain medications in addition to dietary changes will be helpful in preventing recurrence.

Selected Reading

National Kidney Foundation. "Nutrition and chronic kidney disease." www.kidney.org (accessed July 17, 2008).

National Kidney and Urologic Diseases Information Clearinghouse. "Nutrition for Later Chronic Kidney Disease in Adults." http://kidney.niddk.nih.gov/Kudiseases/pubs/NutritionLateCKD/index.htm (accessed on November 2, 2008).

Chapter 4.5

Nutrition and Digestive Problems

Elise M. Brett, MD, MD, FACE, CNSP

The process of normal digestion involves coordinated movements of the various parts of the gastrointestinal tract as well as absorption of nutrients through a healthy intestinal lining. This begins with the breakdown of carbohydrates and fat in the mouth by enzymes found in saliva. The food is then pushed by a part of the throat called the oropharynx into the esophagus, which pushes food further down into the stomach. Protein, fat, and carbohydrates are then broken down by acid and enzymes in the stomach. Stomach movements break apart the food particles into very small pieces. The lower part of the esophagus has a muscular ring, called a sphincter, which tightens and prevents movement of stomach contents back into the esophagus.

The stomach empties into the small intestine. The speed of emptying is partly due to the type of nutrients ingested. Higher fat and fiber-containing foods empty from the stomach more slowly. Most of the nutrient absorption occurs in the small intestine, which is the longest segment of the gastrointestinal tract, measuring 18 to 23 feet. Unabsorbed nutrients, fibers, and food residue then enter the large intestine, called the colon, to prepare for elimination. Undigested fibers are fermented by normal bacteria in the colon, which results in gas production. The colon absorbs water and minerals. The contents that remain are stool, which is eventually eliminated from the body as a bowel movement.

Diet can improve certain gastrointestinal diseases.

Celiac Disease

"Celiac disease," otherwise known as "glutensensitive enteropathy," is a genetic disease in which people have an abnormal response to foods containing the protein "gluten." Ingestion of gluten (contained in grains like wheat, barley, and rye) causes damage to the lining of the intestinal tract so that food cannot be properly absorbed. Diarrhea may or may not be present. Celiac disease that is not treated causes poor absorption of vitamins and minerals, and can lead to iron deficiency anemia and bone loss among other problems.

Complete avoidance of gluten-containing foods usually reverses the intestinal damage. Typical gluten-containing foods include crackers, bread, cereal, cakes, and cookies. However, one must also be aware of hidden sources of gluten found in certain canned soups, salad dressings, ice cream, yogurt, pasta, processed meats, mustard, and ketchup. Even certain medications may contain gluten. Oats may also cause problems for some patients, although it is not clear if this may be due to cross-contamination with wheat in commercially processed oats. Many gluten-free breads, cookies, pastas, and cereals made with substitutes such as rice flour, corn flour, sorghum flour, so flour, cornstarch, and potato starch are now widely available. The key to managing celiac disease is to read food labels carefully in order to avoid gluten. Information about the gluten-free diet and new gluten-free products is also easily available on the Internet (see Suggested Readings below).

Gastroesophageal Reflux

Another gastrointestinal disease that is treated with dietary modification is "gastroesophageal reflux disease," or "GERD." GERD occurs when stomach acid backs up, or refluxes, into the esophagus through the lower esophageal sphincter. This typically causes symptoms of heartburn, a burning sensation in the upper abdomen or chest, but other symptoms such as feeling like the food is sticking, cough, trouble swallowing, voice changes, and worsening asthma can also occur. Over time, GERD can lead to complications such as esophageal stricture, "Barrett's esophagus" (a pre-cancerous condition), and even esophageal cancer.

Some people can be treated with dietary modification, but others require medication to decrease the production or effects of stomach acid. Certain foods have been shown to relax the lower esophageal sphincter and increase reflux. The foods that can worsen symptoms and may need to be limited include fatty foods, fried foods, mint, chocolate, caffeine, tomato, citrus fruits or juices, and alcohol. Spicy foods may also exacerbate symptoms in some people. It is best to decrease overall fat intake and avoid eating large meals. It is often helpful to avoid lying down after eating and avoid eating three hours before bedtime. Obesity also worsens GERD symptoms, and this can be improved with weight loss.

Crohn's Disease

Crohn's disease is a disease that results in inflammation of the intestinal lining. The disease can involve any part of the intestine, and segments in between affected areas may be normal. Symptoms of Crohn's disease may include abdominal pain, diarrhea, intestinal bleeding, fever, and weight loss. Crohn's disease results in periods of flares and periods of inactivity of disease.

There is no evidence that a person's diet causes Crohn's disease, but dietary modification can sometimes be helpful in its treatment. During disease flares, it may be helpful to avoid high fiber foods such as raw fruits, raw vegetables, and beans, which increase gas production and causes belly pain. Nuts and seeds result in increased stool residue and may also make the symptoms worse. White flour products as opposed to whole grains, white rice, plain cereals, crackers, tenderized meat, eggs, potato without the skin, and fruit juices are usually easier to tolerate.

During flares of the disease, it is important to increase fluid and salt intake to avoid dehydration. Commercial products containing high amounts of sodium are available to help maintain fluid and electrolyte balance. Gatorade is not recommended as it contains too much sugar and not enough salt and may even worsen the diarrhea. A home oral rehydration solution can be made by adding 3/4 teaspoon of salt, 4 tablespoons of sugar, 1/2 teaspoon of baking soda, and 1/2 teaspoon of 20 percent potassium chloride solution to one liter of water. Additional flavoring can be added for improved taste. Sometimes, intravenous nutrition (TPN) may become necessary during disease flares to rest the bowel (see chapter 4.11, "Artificial Nutrition").

During periods of disease inactivity, a usual healthy diet is recommended without specific restrictions. Probiotics are live bacteria that are designed to improve intestinal bacterial balance.

Ingesting certain probiotics has been shown to help maintain remission in some people with Crohn's disease.

Irritable bowel syndrome

Irritable bowel syndrome (IBS) is a common gastrointestinal disorder. IBS is diagnosed when recurrent symptoms of abdominal pain or distension are associated with a change in frequency or consistency of bowel movements, in the absence of other gastrointestinal disease. Symptoms of IBS are often relieved by a bowel movement.

Persons with IBS may have certain food sensitivities. Eliminating certain foods from the diet and rotating foods that cause symptoms every few days has been shown to be helpful in some patients. True food allergies have not yet been clearly identified but are being studied and may prove to be important in IBS (see chapter 4.14, "Food Allergies"). Some of the most common food intolerances are lactose, wheat products, and monosaccharides such as sorbitol and fructose. Keeping a food and symptom diary can be helpful in managing the disorder. Any food that is consistently associated with symptoms should be avoided in the future.

Altered intestinal bacteria may also play a role in causing symptoms in people with IBS. Treatment with probiotics has been shown to improve symptoms in some research studies, but the results are inconsistent. Interestingly, peppermint oil relaxes the smooth muscle of the intestine and has been shown in several research studies to relieve symptoms of IBS. The effect of fiber on irritable bowel syndrome has been studied and has not been shown to result in clear benefit. Although fiber intake is often recommended by practitioners for people with constipation, gas production by fermentation of fiber in the colon may actually worsen symptoms. Increasing fiber intake modestly, by 2 to 3 grams a day, may be an approach worth trying. Certain eating habits are associated with the inadvertent swallowing of air, which can form intestinal gas and cause pain. When this is a problem, one should avoid eating large meals, especially very quickly (it is better to eat smaller meals and eat more slowly), drink adequate amounts of water (six to eight 8-ounce glasses a day), avoid carbonated beverages or sodas, and avoid chewing gum.

Suggested Readings

Celiac Sprue Association. http://www.csaceliacs.org/gluten_grains.php (accessed on August 31, 2008).

Crohn's and Colitis Foundation. "Diet and Nutrition." http://www.ccfa.org/info/diet?LMI=4.2 (accessed on August 31, 2008).

Gluten-free.com. http://www.glutenfree.com/ (accessed on August 31, 2008).

Medline Plus. "GERD." http://www.nlm.nih.gov/medlineplus/gerd.html (accessed on August 31, 2008).

National Digestive Diseases Information Clearing House (NDDIC). "Heartburn, Gastroesophageal Reflux (GER), and Gastroesophageal Reflux Disease (GERD)." http://digestive.niddk.nih.gov/ddiseases/pubs/gerd/ (accessed on August 31, 2008).

National Digestive Diseases Information Clearing House (NDDIC). "Irritable Bowel Syndrome." http://digestive.niddk.nih.gov/ddiseases/pubs/ibs/ (accessed on August 31, 2008).

Chapter 4.6

Nutrition and Blood Fats: Beyond Cholesterol

Maria L. Collazo-Clavell, MD

Heart disease remains the number one cause of death for both men and women in the United States. Most people have heard about how high cholesterol levels in the blood can increase one's chance of developing a heart attack. However, other types of blood fats, or "lipids," are also important.

What Are These Blood Fats?

Blood fats include triglycerides, high-density lipoprotein (HDL) cholesterol (a "good" cholesterol), and the total cholesterol, which is mostly made up of a "bad" cholesterol called low-density lipoprotein, or "LDL"-cholesterol. Although it can be measured directly, LDL is generally calculated by using the values of the three measurements in an arithmetic formula:

LDL = TOTAL CHOLESTEROL – HDL – TRIGLYCERIDES / 5.

So, if the total cholesterol is 200, the HDL is 40, and the triglycerides are 150, then the LDL is "200 minus 40 minus 30," which equals 130.

LDL is the main culprit that increases the chance for heart disease by promoting cholesterol deposits in the blood vessels and blocking the flow of blood. In general, the higher the LDL level, the greater the chance for blockages to develop. HDL is the good cholesterol because it acts to reverse this process. HDL can remove cholesterol deposits from the blood vessels and protect against blockages. The higher the HDL, the greater the protection against heart disease. Triglycerides are another blood fat that can carry LDL and promote cholesterol deposits in the blood vessels. However, triglycerides can cause blockages of the blood vessels in other ways, such as making the blood clot more easily. It is important to understand that the cholesterol levels in your bloodstream result from cholesterol in the foods you eat and from production by your body (see figure, page 144).

How Can I Protect Myself against Heart Disease?

Keeping blood fats in a good range has been shown to protect against heart disease. That means trying to keep total cholesterol, LDL, and triglycerides low and HDL high. However, blood fats are only part of the equation. How low LDL needs to be depends on an individual's risk factors for heart disease. The more risk factors for heart disease there are, the lower LDL should be. So, if there is a history of smoking, diabetes, hypertension, or a family history of heart disease, it is advised that LDL be lower than if those risk factors were absent (table 1). Additionally, an HDL greater than 60 is thought to protect against heart disease.

What Affects Blood Fats?

Many things contribute to LDL, HDL, and triglyceride levels. Genes that are inherited from one's parents can affect the levels of blood fats by determining how they are produced and removed from the blood. Eating habits, such as eating foods with high amounts of fat or sugar, can raise the cholesterol and triglyceride levels in the blood. If a person is overweight or obese, the cholesterol and triglyceride levels may be increased since the body's ability to remove these fats from the blood is impaired. A person's activity level can also affect blood fats. If a person is inactive, LDL and triglycerides may be increased because there is decreased removal of these fats from the bloodstream. In addition, HDL is decreased. A person's age is also important. As one grows older, LDL and triglycerides tend to rise, especially in women after menopause. Gender affects blood fats. Estrogen (the female sex hormone) and testosterone (the male sex hormone) affect blood fats differently. Estrogen tends to increase the HDL and can protect against heart disease before menopause. Testosterone can lower the HDL, increasing the risk for heart disease. This difference between men and women is the main reason why men tend to develop heart disease at a younger age.

Finally, alcohol intake can affect blood fat levels. Too much alcohol intake can increase triglyceride levels and damage the liver. However, moderate amounts of alcohol intake, one (women) or two (men) servings of beer, wine, or spirits per day, can increase the HDL and possibly decrease the risk for heart disease. However, this observation, which has been used to explain many of the "health benefits" of alcohol, should not be misinterpreted. Irresponsible alcohol consumption can lead to increased use in certain people, absenteeism from work, and motor vehicle accidents. Therefore, people who drink too much alcohol should decrease their consumption to at least moderate levels, if not less. More importantly, there is *insufficient strong evidence* to recommend that people should increase their consumption of alcohol in order to be healthier. To repeat: people should *not* increase alcohol consumption to be healthy.

What Dietary Changes Can Improve Blood Fats?

Although there are many dietary recommendations available, they all share the same principles when it comes to the prevention of heart disease.

1. Limit the intake of fat. It is recommended that only 30 percent of total calories in the diet come from fat. That means that if someone follows a 1,500-calorie-a-day diet, less than 500 calories should come from fat. This would be less than 55 grams of fat a day.
2. Limit the intake of saturated fats. Saturated fats are particularly bad, and it is recommended that they be limited to less than 10 percent of total calories. If we use the

same example of a 1,500-calorie-a-day diet, only 150 calories should be from saturated fats, or less than 17 grams of saturated fat for each day. Replacing saturated fats with "monounsaturated" and "polyunsaturated" fats can help lower LDL-cholesterol (see chapter 2.2, "Fats" and chapter 5.1, "Biochemistry of Nutrition" for explanations on monounsaturated and polyunsaturated fats).

3. Avoid *trans* fats. *Trans* fats are created when hydrogen is added to vegetable oil. *Trans* fats may be used in many prepackaged foods such as crackers and cookies. Recent studies suggest that *trans* fats increase the risk for heart disease.
4. Limit the intake of dietary cholesterol if it is too much. It is recommended that the daily intake of cholesterol be limited to less than 300 milligrams per day. Sometimes, especially in the setting of heart disease, lower amounts such as less than 200 milligrams per day are recommended. These recommendations may change in the future as more scientific information becomes available about the impact of dietary cholesterol on health risks.
5. Increase the intake of high-fiber foods. Most high-fiber foods are low in fat and cholesterol. A high-fiber diet can also lower cholesterol.
6. Limit the intake of sodium. It is recommended that healthy adults limit their intake of sodium to 1,500 to 2,400 milligrams per day.
7. Control the intake of calories. Controlling the intake of excess calories helps people better manage their weight. Being overweight or obese increases the chances of having high levels of cholesterol and triglycerides in the blood, increases blood sugar, and increases blood pressure. All of these effects will increase the chances for a heart attack.

How Does One Introduce These Changes into a Daily Routine?

1. Limit the intake of fat. Foods high in fat tend to be animal products or plant oils. To lower the intake of high-fat foods:
   - Choose lean meats such as chicken and turkey. As an example, ground turkey can replace ground beef when making a pasta meat sauce.
   - Avoid frying; opt for baking, broiling, or grilling.
   - Introduce one meat-less meal per week and then even more meat-less meals per week if you can.
   - Make one night a "salad night." Family members can even make their own individual salads. Tear or chop up a leaf lettuce and cut up lots of colorful vegetables such as carrots, tomatoes, cucumbers, bell peppers, and red onions for toppings. Beans, low-fat cheeses, or sliced grilled chicken breast can be added to provide protein. Nuts, but not to excess, may be incorporated since they tend to be high in monounsaturated fats. Use a low-fat or olive oil-based dressing, preferably without mayonnaise.

2. Limit the intake of saturated fats. Saturated fats are also found in animal products, such as butter and lard. Replacing saturated fats with monounsaturated and polyunsaturated fats can help control cholesterol. Monounsaturated fats are found in olive, canola, and peanut oils, avocados, and many nuts. Polyunsaturated fats are

found in sunflower, corn, and soy oils. Butter, which contains saturated animal fat, should be used sparingly or substituted when preparing recipes. Many times, butter can be replaced by olive oil.

3. Avoid *trans* fats. Food manufacturers are required to list the amount of *trans* fats in food labels. Therefore, the Nutrition Facts Label should be reviewed when shopping at the food market (see chapter 1.2).
4. Limit the intake of cholesterol. Animal products are the main source of cholesterol in the diet. However, limiting does not mean doing without.

   - Decrease the number and frequency of eggs or eliminate just the cholesterol-containing yolks if you are consuming too much cholesterol. Try boiled or poached eggs to avoid additional fat in preparation, such as butter or margarine used for frying.
   - Limit the use of butter and mayonnaise. Choose spreads such as peanut butter on toast or even olive oil and vinegar on a sandwich.
   - Choose lower fat alternatives for milk, cheese, and yogurt. No-fat or lower fat alternatives are always better options. It is recommended that people choose foods with less than 5 grams of fat per serving.

5. Increase the intake of high-fiber foods. Foods high in fiber are fruits, vegetables, oats, whole grains, and beans.

   - Choose whole-grain breads and pastas.
   - Replace breadcrumbs with oats in a favorite meat loaf.
   - Find recipes for bean soups and salads.
   - Always have fresh fruit around for a healthy snack.

6. Limit the intake of sodium. Foods high in sodium include prepackaged foods such as soups, canned vegetables, luncheon meats, and frozen meals. Meals prepared outside of the home also tend to be high in sodium.

   - Limit eating out and purchasing prepackaged foods.
   - Limit salt added during food preparation.
   - Try other spices instead of salt, such as garlic, oregano, or basil.

7. Control the intake of calories. Remember, following a lower fat diet does not necessarily mean eating fewer calories. Be careful with food labels advertising low-fat foods since they often replace fat calories with calories from other sources.

What If These Changes Are Too Hard to Do?

Change is always hard and requires effort. It is best to pace one's self by setting goals that can be achieved. One option is to seek help from a registered dietitian to learn how to go about improving eating habits. One should not be discouraged if it takes longer than he or she thought to incorporate dietary change. It is important to be supportive of family members who are trying to implement dietary changes.

Suggested Readings

American Association of Clinical Endocrinologists. "Power of Prevention, Endocrine Health, cholesterol." http://www.powerofprevention.com/cholesterol.php (accessed on September 21, 2008).

American Heart Association. "Cholesterol." http://www.americanheart.org/presenter.jhtml?identifier=1516 (accessed on September 21, 2008).

Centers for Disease Control and Prevention. "Nutrition for Everyone, dietary fat." http://www.cdc.gov/nccdphp/dnpa/nutrition/nutrition_for_everyone/basics/fat.htm (accessed on September 21, 2008).

Learn more about eggs. http://www.aeb.org/LearnMore/EggsGoodHealth.htm (accessed on September 21, 2008).

Mayoclinic.com. "Dietary Fats." http://www.mayoclinic.com/health/fat/NU00262 (accessed on September 21, 2008).

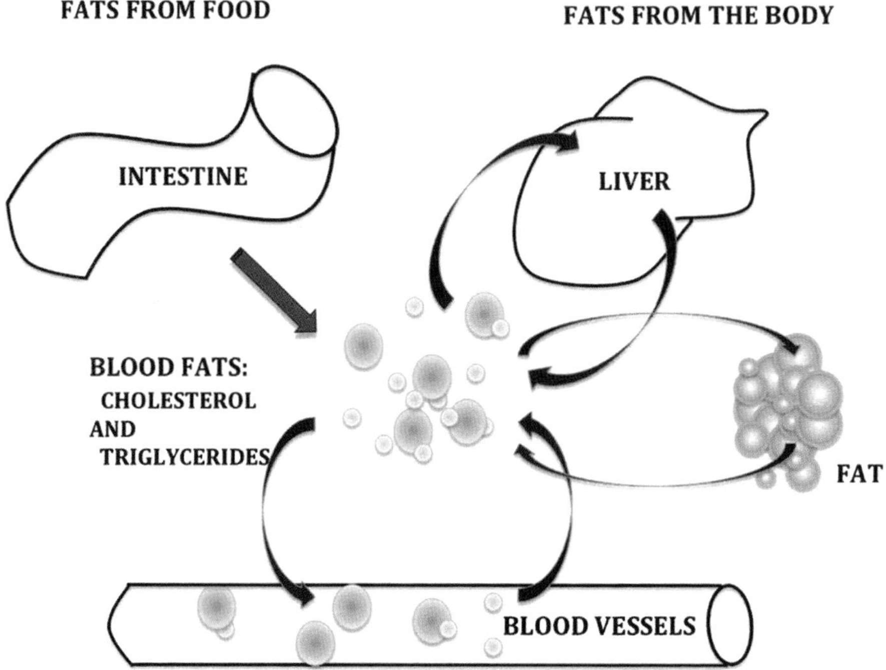

Blood fats are from the food we eat and also made in our body (see text, page 139).

Table. Risk factors for heart disease and desired cholesterol levels

Number of Risk Factors	Desired LDL cholesterol Level (mg/dL)
0	<160
1	<130
>2 OR presence of diabetes	<100 (consider <70)

Risk factors are are >55 years (men) or >65 years (women), smoking, hypertnesion, family history of heart disease for a male family member (<45 years) or female family member (< years). Triglyceride levels should be <150 mg/dL while HDL cholesterol desired goal is > 40 mg/dL.

Chapter 4.7

Nutrition and Heart Disease

Jeffrey I. Mechanick, MD, FACP, FACE, FACN

There is perhaps no health issue more apparent to Americans than the prevention of a heart attack. A heart attack causes acute pain, can be life-threatening, and can lead to heart damage, which can quickly limit a person's ability to perform ordinary activities. Heart disease is costly also. Medical costs associated with a chronically ill person can negatively impact a family's quality of life as well as have an enormous financial burden on the country as a whole.

It is oversimplified to say that heart attacks occur because we eat poorly, do not really exercise enough, and are under far too much stress. There is clearly a genetic component to our risk to develop heart disease, and despite the many complicated biochemical and molecular reasons for heart attacks, it is still fair to say that our eating habits affect our chances of having heart disease. Nevertheless, despite plenty of media coverage on the risks for heart attacks with unhealthy eating and the personal stories from friends and families about the tremendous burdens of chronic illness, there are still shortcomings in healthy eating practices.

What are the dietary risk factors associated with heart disease? Heart attacks result from clogging of the arteries that supply precious oxygen and nutrients to the heart. Clogging of the heart, or "coronary," arteries is due to inflammation of the blood vessel wall. Many factors can contribute to this process, like too much bad cholesterol ("LDL-cholesterol") in the bloodstream, high blood pressure, high blood sugar as seen with diabetes, and being overweight or obese. Here is a list of nutrients that when consumed too much may lead to an *increased* risk of heart attacks:

- Saturated fats (saturated fatty acids [SFA]; mainly animal fats and tropical oils: palm and coconut)
- Cholesterol (also an animal fat in meats, dairy, and egg yolk)
- *Trans* fatty acids (frequently found in "fast" foods, especially french fries and donuts, and "stick" margarine but not "soft-tub" margarine)

On the other hand, here is a list of nutrients that when consumed instead of the high-risk foods above can lead to a *decreased* risk of heart disease:

- Monounsaturated fatty acids (MUFA; found in olive, canola, and peanut oils and avocados)
- Polyunsaturated fatty acids (PUFA; including safflower, sesame, soy, corn, and sunflower

oils, seeds, and nuts, like walnuts, almonds, pecans)
- Omega-3 fatty acids (n-3 FA; found in cold-water fish such as mackerel, salmon, herring, trout, sardines, and tuna)
- Fiber (found in fresh fruits, fresh vegetables, and whole grains)
- Plant stanols/sterols (also found in margarine, orange juice, yogurt, some cereals, and nuts: walnuts, almonds, pecans; these compounds decrease dietary cholesterol absorption from the intestine)
- Soy protein (as a beneficial protein source, instead of high SFA protein sources such as red meats)

Current recommendations to reduce the risk of heart disease are to reduce SFA to less than 7 to 10 percent total calories for the day and cholesterol to less than 200 to 300 milligrams for the day, depending on the severity of the risk reduction needed. Strategies to limit the SFA content of meat consumed include: limiting the serving size to just 3 ounces (½ chicken breast, ¾ cup of flaked fish, or 2 thin slices of lean roast beef: 3" x 3" x ¼"); choosing lean cuts of meat; preparing meats by braising, broiling, roasting, or stir-frying (not deep-frying); removing skin and visible fat before preparation; limiting organ meats (for example, liver) to once a month; and skimming off fat when preparing gravies, soups, or stews. When cooking or baking, one can choose a fat source that is relatively lower in SFA. The SFA, MUFA, PUFA, and cholesterol contents of various oils and fats are given in the table below.

Table. Amount of Saturated and Unsaturated Fat by Type of Oil or Fat

Type of oil or fat	%SFA	%MUFA	%PUFA	Cholesterol (grams/L)
Canola oil	6	62	31	0
Safflower oil	9	12	78	0
Sunflower oil	11	20	69	0
Corn oil	13	25	62	0
Peanut oil	13	49	33	0
Olive oil	14	77	9	0
Soybean oil	15	24	61	0
Margarine	18	48	29	0
Vegetable shortening	25	43	25	0
Cottonseed oil	27	19	54	0
Chicken fat	30	47	22	2.2
Lard	41	47	12	2.4
Animal fat shortening	43	48	6	1.8
Beef fat	51	44	4	2.8
Palm oil	51	39	10	0
Butter	54	30	12	6.6
Coconut oil	77	6	15	0

A healthy eating plan should include more than 25 to 30 grams of fiber (with greater than 7–13 grams of soluble fiber) a day. *Trans* fats should be less than 1 percent of all calories consumed, or completely avoided. The use of soy or other oils rich in MUFA/PUFA is recommended. Meals should contain other healthy foods including fresh fruits and vegetables (more than 8–10 servings a day) and whole grains instead of processed flour and starches. Adding unsalted nuts to the meal instead of sugary or starchy foods is also a good idea. The Dietary Approaches to Stop Hypertension, or "DASH," diet consists largely of fresh fruits, fresh vegetables, and low-fat dairy products. This diet is relatively low in sodium and high in potassium. Oily fish, more than two 4-ounce servings per week, or up to 3 grams of n-3 FA per day, is also recommended.

Other dietary factors are still being studied. Caffeine, found in coffee, tea, and chocolate, affects the heart, but it is still not clear whether it is truly bad for you. Moderation is the best approach, and limiting coffee to 1 to 2 cups per day is prudent. Small amounts (around 3 ounces a day) of dark chocolate have also been associated with benefit in terms of lowering the risk of heart disease. However, the downsides to regular consumption of chocolate are dental cavities, increased calories, and kidney stones from the oxalate content.

Alcohol consumption is still a controversial issue because there are some effects of alcohol and other chemicals (resveratrol and flavonoids, for example) in red wine that may reduce the risk of heart disease. However, the current scientific evidence supports a position that if you do not drink alcohol regularly, do not to start. The risks of motor vehicle accidents, addiction (alcoholism), high blood pressure, obesity, stroke, and suicide due to the effects of alcohol outweigh any proven benefits. Also, people who have high triglyceride levels, are overweight or obese, or already have heart disease or hypertension should severely limit alcohol. People with diabetes may be at increased risk for low blood sugar when drinking alcohol. Women who are pregnant should not drink alcohol. Other people who enjoy drinking should limit alcohol consumption to below one beverage a day for women or two beverages a day for men. One beverage serving of alcohol (120–180 calories per serving) is:

- 0.5 ounces (15 grams) pure grain alcohol
- 12 ounces (355 milliliter) beer
- 5 ounces (148 milliliter) wine
- 1.5 ounces (44 milliliter) 80-proof distilled spirits
- 1 ounce (30 milliliter) 100-proof distilled spirits.
- Various antioxidants have been studied with respect to the prevention of heart disease.

However, no conclusive studies favor the routine use of any vitamins or other dietary supplements with antioxidant properties for the prevention or treatment of heart disease. A diet rich in foods that contain compounds with antioxidant properties, such as a plant-based diet with fresh fruits and vegetables, along with unsalted nuts, whole grains, low- or non-fat dairy products, oils with MUFA and PUFA, and oily fish as a protein source, would be a sensible strategy for healthy eating to prevent heart disease. Naturally, this should be accompanied by a daily physical activity program, maintenance of a healthy weight, blood pressure control with a low (less than 2,300 milligrams per day) sodium diet, prevention and proper treatment of diabetes, treatment of any lipid (high cholesterol and/or high triglyceride) problems, proper amounts of sleep, and stress reduction. This approach is what we call a "healthy lifestyle."

Selected Reading

American Heart Association. "Our 2006 diet and lifestyle recommendations." www.americanheart.org (accessed July 17, 2008).

Texas Heart Institute. "Nutrition." http://www.texasheart.org/HIC/Topics/HSmart/nutriti1.cfm (accessed on November 2, 2008).

US Department of Agriculture. "Diet and Disease, heart health." http://fnic.nal.usda.gov/nal_display/index.php?info_center=4&tax_level=2&tax_subject=278&topic_id=1378 (accessed on November 2, 2008).

Chapter 4.8

Nutrition and Cancer

Jeffrey I. Mechanick, MD, FACP, FACE, FACN

Introduction

Cancer is a medical term that is used to describe diseases that result from uncontrolled growth of abnormal cells, which can invade normal tissues. This creates of a state of inflammation and tissue damage that can potentially lead to death. Some cancers are for the most part "curable," like some skin cancers, most types of thyroid cancers and prostate cancers, early breast cancer, childhood leukemia, testicular cancer, and Hodgkin's disease, to name a few. Unfortunately, other cancers are extremely difficult to treat, and new treatment strategies are constantly sought out.

The way in which cancers behave, particularly the way they behave differently in different people, is due to hereditary factors and environmental factors. Certain nutritional factors have long been implicated as important environmental components in the prevention of various cancers and their successful treatment. Other environmental factors that have been shown to play a role in inducing cancer are tobacco smoking, toxic chemical exposure, and radiation exposure. These factors are called "carcinogens." In addition to the ways in which nutrition affects cancer prevention and treatment, a healthy eating program and maintenance of normal weight are also important to speed recovery.

Nutrition and Cancer Prevention

It is thought that up to 30 to 40 percent of all cancers are in some fashion linked to poor dietary habits; this number may be as high as 70 percent for cancers involving the gastrointestinal tract. For example, a high intake of nitrite-cured foods, such as hot dogs, bacon, ham, and salt-cured fish, has been linked to cancers of the stomach, esophagus, and pancreas. These foods should be eaten in limited quantities.

A key element of how foods can prevent cancer is related to "phytochemicals" (chemicals found in plants). Many scientific studies have supported the finding that plant-based diets, compared with those having minimal fruits and vegetables and lots of meat, starch, sugar, and saturated fat, are associated with a lower risk of cancer. Besides the studies that have shown that eating a lot of fruits or vegetables of varying types can decrease all types of cancer, benefits have been specifically attributed to raw vegetables, cruciferous vegetables (such as broccoli, cauliflower, cabbage, and brussels sprouts), allium vegetables (such as garlic, onions, and shallots), green vegetables, tomatoes, and citrus fruits. The strongest evidence of fruits and vegetables having a preventive effect is for stomach, esophagus, large intestine, mouth, throat, and lung cancers. Weaker evidence is also available for voice box (larynx), pancreas, breast, bladder, ovary, uterus, cervix, thyroid, prostate, kidney, and liver cancers.

How do phytochemicals prevent cancer? There are several mechanisms that are supported by scientific studies, though sufficient information from clinical studies with real people is limited:

- Free radical scavenging to decrease damage to genetic material ("DNA") and prevent accumulation of genetic mutations (isothiocyanates in cruciferous vegetables; beta-carotene, vitamins A and C in many fruits and vegetables; selenium in meats)
- Inducing programmed cell death ("apoptosis") of precancer or cancer cells before they become too dangerous (curcumin in turmeric; resveratrol from grapes and red wine)
- Preventing the way in which cancer cells stimulate blood vessels to form; a group of cancer cells that spreads throughout the body by way of the bloodstream is called a "metastasis" (epigallocatechin-3-gallate [EGCG] in green tea and dark chocolate; ellagic acid in raspberries and strawberries; delphinidin in blueberries)
- Preventing the inflammatory response that helps cancers progress (curcumin and resveratrol)

Does this information mean that we should all flock to the corner pharmacy or health food store to buy dietary supplements containing these ingredients? No, but it does mean that there may be some healthy choices available in the form of whole foods that may offer some cancer prevention attributes without the risks of potent dietary supplements and potential interactions of dietary supplements with medications (see chapter 4.12, "Dietary Supplements").

The following is a brief summary of dietary strategies associated with reduced risk for cancer.

- Eat plenty of fresh fruits and vegetables.
- Eat enough fiber.
- Limit red meat and saturated fats.
- Maintain a normal body weight—not undernourished and not overweight or obese.
- Limit or avoid alcohol.
- Avoid contaminated foods or foods exposed to environmental carcinogens.
- Limit nitrite-cured foods.

Nutrition and Cancer Treatment

Fifty percent of cancer patients have poor nutritional status and unintentional weight loss at the time of their diagnosis. This is due to (1) "anorexia" or loss of appetite, which can be related to altered taste or smell or the inflammatory condition that accompanies many cancers; (2) problems with the gastrointestinal tract that result from decreased nutrient absorption, obstruction so food cannot pass through, early feelings of fullness, or chronic nausea and vomiting; and/or (3) accelerated tissue breakdown also due to inflammation.

Undernutrition can have a negative effect on the response to cancer treatment. Sometimes, cancer patients are overweight or obese at the time of diagnosis, and this is also a metabolic disadvantage. While it is still not entirely clear whether being overweight or obese has a direct negative effect on a person's response to cancer treatment, it can have an indirect negative impact on their overall survival. Therefore, any patient with a nutritional disorder prior to cancer treatment should seek out specialized counseling, preferably by a physician experienced with nutritional disorders or a registered dietitian (RD).

During cancer treatment, nutritional status can worsen. This is due to side effects of chemotherapy, radiation therapy, and surgical therapy on taste, smell, and the gastrointestinal tract, as well as effects from chronic pain, depression, anxiety, and confusion. The goals of nutritional therapy during cancer treatment are to maintain a normal weight, correct any nutritional deficiencies that may develop, and treat the adverse effects of the cancer treatment that are compromising the nutritional status.

In fact, improvement of the nutritional status during cancer treatment improves a person's overall quality of life and ability to perform tasks of everyday life. For instance, if decreased appetite is the problem, then the patient should try to consume smaller meals, more frequently. Choosing foods that have a high caloric density and taste good is another approach. Examples are ice cream, shakes, mashed potatoes, and ground beef, but different people will have different preferences.

Frequently, chemotherapy patients have sore mouths right after a treatment, and Italian ices, sherbets, and ice creams can be soothing. During this time of discomfort, it may not be possible to meet nutritional needs, which is why more food is needed between treatments when symptoms are less. In cases where nutritional needs cannot be met for a period of time more than just a few days, other strategies need to be used. Nutritional supplements are available over-the-counter, and a doctor or RD can make recommendations. These products have different tastes and caloric densities, so some variety is possible and some may be better tolerated than others.

If nutritional intake remains poor for more than several weeks and weight loss is becoming a more serious problem, a doctor may recommend one of two forms of nutrition support. The first type of nutrition support is "enteral" nutrition, or "tube feeds." This is when a soft tube is placed down the nose into the stomach or intestine ("nasogastric" or "nasoenteric" feeding tube) or a soft tube is placed directly through the skin into the stomach or intestine ("percutaneous endoscopic gastrostomy," or "PEG"; "percutaneous endoscopic jejunostomy," or "PEJ"; surgically placed gastrostomy; surgically placed jejunostomy). Liquid feedings can provide all the calories, protein, vitamins, and minerals that are needed when given in sufficient quantities.

Sometimes, a person cannot tolerate adequate enteral nutrition. In a second type of nutrition support, nutrition is provided "parenterally," or directly into the bloodstream. This is commonly referred to as "TPN," or "total parenteral nutrition," and generally requires the placement of a special intravenous catheter, called a "central line." This intravenous catheter can be inserted into one of the larger veins in the neck or upper arm. The latter type in the upper arm is called a "peripherally-inserted central catheter," or "PICC." If parenteral nutrition is required or anticipated for many weeks to months during cancer treatment, as when there is an obstruction of the gastrointestinal tract, TPN can even be given at home. (For a more detailed discussion of enteral and parenteral nutrition, see chapter 4.11, "Artificial Nutrition.")

Dietary supplements have been discussed above in terms of cancer prevention, and the point was made that consuming a plant-based diet, rich in antioxidants, was recommended over the injudicious consumption of over-the-counter products advertised as beneficial. The same is generally true for the use of dietary supplements during cancer treatment. Some of these dietary supplements studied during cancer treatment in animal experiments and limited human trials include: L-carnitine, polyunsaturated and omega-3 fatty acids, RNA and DNA, polyphenols, alpha-lipoic acid, and vitamin E.

While the theoretical advantages of certain dietary supplements cannot be refuted, their clear benefit and safety with cancer treatment in humans is generally unproven. Any exceptions to this rule, and there are some, must be discussed and approved by the treating physician. This is because there are still some practical issues with dietary supplements and cancer treatment:

- Just because a particular dietary supplement is proven beneficial and safe in one or more studies does not mean it will help all patients with the disease.
- Many dietary supplements interfere with the beneficial activity of the primary cancer treatment, like folate and methotrexate (a chemotherapy that deliberately interferes with folate metabolism), or antioxidants and chemo-/radio-therapy in which oxidative damage to cancer cells is desired.
- Many dietary supplement doses may exceed what is safe.
- The amount and type (quality control) of a particular brand of dietary supplement is frequently different from what the label indicates or what the purchaser wants and may even contain contaminants.

Nutrition and Cancer Recovery

For survivors of cancer treatment, there is a need to reestablish a healthy lifestyle. This consists of basically the same principles that apply for non-cancer patients. Any deviations will need to be discussed with your cancer doctor. In general, a healthy lifestyle after cancer treatment involves:

- Healthy eating
  - Maintain a normal body weight (do not overcompensate by regaining weight above what is normal)
  - Eat a plant-based diet
  - 8 to 10 or even more servings of fresh fruits and vegetables per day
  - 25 to 30 grams of fiber per day
  - Limited saturated fats, sugary and starchy foods
  - Use of monounsaturated or polyunsaturated cooking oils (olive, canola, sunflower, and safflower)
  - Plenty of whole grains, legumes (beans, peas, and lentils), and nuts
  - More fish and poultry and limited red meat; when eating red meats, make sure they are lean
  - Use low-fat or no-fat dairy products
  - Take precautions when eating out—try to stick to a healthy eating plan

- Regular physical activity
  - Build up to a structured exercise program of at least thirty to sixty minutes per day
  - Use the stairs instead of the elevator
  - Walk more instead of using cars, buses, trains, or subways

- Adequate sleep
- Stress reduction

An unfortunate reality about cancer is that some patients do not survive. In this situation, a declining nutritional status is more of an indicator of advanced cancer than a cause of subsequent poor functional status. In this terminal phase of cancer, in which "cachexia" (loss of body mass that includes muscle mass and fat mass) is often apparent, nutrition support rarely has benefit and may even introduce additional risks. Even though many terminally ill cancer patients cannot eat or drink sufficiently, they can consume enough food for comfort. Nevertheless, there are still concerns by family, friends, and even some doctors whether a more aggressive approach to nutrition in this setting is needed. One approach that is generally accepted is to continue to "offer" food and water to the terminally ill cancer patient but to refrain from using aggressive nutrition support if there is no hope of benefit. Obviously, there are many factors that contribute to difficult decisions such as withholding nutrition support, so having a frank discussion with the treating doctor is necessary.

Suggested Reading

American Cancer Society. "Nutrition for the Person with Cancer." http://www.cancer.org/docroot/MBC/MBC_6.asp (accessed on November 2, 2008).

National Cancer Institute. "Overview of Nutrition in Cancer Care." http://www.cancer.gov/cancerinfo/pdq/supportivecare/nutrition (accessed on November 2, 2008).

University of Texas, M.D. Anderson Cancer Center. "Nutrition and Cancer." http://www.mdanderson.org/topics/food/ (accessed on November 2, 2008).

Chapter 4.9

Nutrition and Bone Health

Donald Bergman, MD

Introduction

The ad gets your attention—a celebrity with a "milk mustache" tells you that milk keeps you healthy and builds strong bones. From birth until the teenage years, we follow the advice in the milk advertisement and get an adequate amount of milk and milk products. Most people then lose a taste for milk and start drinking soda and caffeinated beverages such as coffee and tea. This results in a lack of calcium in the diet, which leads to a gradual wearing away of bone and, along with osteoporosis (an inherited disorder of bone), can lead to deformity of the spine and fracture of the hips and long bones.

People who are calcium deficient are also likely to be vitamin D deficient. There is very little vitamin D in our diets. Most dietary vitamin D comes from certain fish oils, such as cod liver oil, and from vitamin D-fortified milk. We need vitamin D to help with calcium absorption. Most of the vitamin D we need is made in our skin by exposure to sunlight. However, we avoid sunlight or use sunscreen because of concern about skin cancer. As a result, we become vitamin D deficient and must be aware of our need to consume more foods and supplements with vitamin D.

Calcium Metabolism

What Does Calcium Do?

Calcium accounts for about 2 percent of an adult's body weight. Ninety-nine percent of the calcium is found in bone and teeth, and the rest is in blood and inside each cell. Calcium combines with phosphorus and forms a crystal, which is deposited within bone. This calcium phosphate crystal is deposited and scattered in small amounts throughout bone collagen (like the collagen that is found in and under your skin). This arrangement allows bone to be hard (due to the calcium crystals) and yet very flexible (due to the bone collagen) at the same time.

As important as calcium is to the structure of bone, calcium serves even more important functions in the rest of the body. Calcium serves as a signal when it moves from the blood into and around the cells of the body. This movement of calcium causes muscles to contract, blood vessels to constrict, and nerves to transmit signals. Calcium is also important for blood clotting and for the release of hormones. These functions of calcium are so important that, if you are not consuming enough calcium in the diet, the body will dissolve bone to release calcium to the rest of the body, causing the bones to become thin and increasing the risk of fracture.

How Do I Increase the Calcium I Eat?

There are many good sources of dietary calcium. Dairy products, many nuts and seeds, some fish, particularly salmon and sardines (canned with the bones), figs, tofu and other soybean products, and some vegetables such as beans, kale, and seaweed are good sources of calcium. A few foods, such as rhubarb, collard greens, and mustard greens, are high in calcium also but contain other chemicals that may decrease calcium absorption.

If one does not get enough calcium through food, then it is possible to take calcium supplements. The major types of calcium available are calcium carbonate, calcium phosphate, and calcium citrate. There is more calcium per tablet in the calcium carbonate and calcium phosphate than in the calcium citrate, but the carbonate and phosphate forms of calcium require more stomach acid for their absorption than the citrate. As we get older, we make less acid, so citrate is the preferred form for older individuals. The exception is older individuals who have kidney failure. They need a different form of calcium and should check with their physicians. Calcium carbonate should be taken with meals because there is more stomach acid secreted during a meal.

It is important not to take medicine at the same time as calcium, since the calcium can interfere with the absorption of certain medications. Read the label carefully on the bottle. The label may indicate the amount of calcium carbonate per tablet (1,250 milligrams, for example), but calcium carbonate is only 40 percent calcium (meaning that there is only 500 milligrams of actual calcium per tablet in our example). Calcium citrate is only 20 percent calcium. The label should state how much calcium each tablet contains (sometimes called "elemental calcium" on the label). If this is not clearly stated, a pharmacist can help calculate how much calcium is provided.

Certain things can interfere with maintaining a good level of calcium. Phosphorus is one. Calcium and phosphorus are necessary for healthy bones and teeth, but foods that are high in phosphorus and low in calcium, such as artificially carbonated soda, may slightly lower calcium levels in the blood. This causes the body to dissolve bone to keep the blood calcium normal. Although strong evidence for this is lacking, it is wise to balance soft drink consumption with reliable sources of calcium.

Sodium in the diet can cause the body to lose calcium in the urine. It is not clear how important this is with ordinary salt intake, but it is a good idea to avoid excess salt in the diet. Diuretics can also affect calcium balance. Diuretics are often referred to as "water pills" and are generally prescribed by doctors to help reduce body water by increasing urination. Diuretics called "loop diuretics" can cause loss of calcium in the urine, while diuretics called "thiazide diuretics" can reduce calcium losses. Thiazide diuretics can occasionally lead to an abnormally high level of calcium in the blood. Drugs that are used to treat heartburn and ulcers by decreasing stomach acid have also been shown to decrease bone mass. It is not clear whether this type of drug causes decreased calcium absorption, but calcium intake and bone density should be carefully monitored in people taking stomach acid-lowering drugs.

The recommended intake of calcium (dietary and supplements combined) for adults is about 1,000-1,200 milligrams daily. Other people, such as those with certain medical illnesses or on certain medications, may need more or less than 1,200 milligrams of calcium a day. If you have any concerns about your calcium intake, you should discuss this with your doctor.

Sometimes, your doctor will ask you to collect a urine sample for calcium over a twenty-four-hour period to determine the right amount of calcium intake.

Is It Possible to Consume Too Much Calcium?

There are some negatives about calcium supplementation; some reports have surfaced suggesting an increased risk of prostate cancer and heart attack. Other studies have reported just the opposite. Until more data becomes available, taking the recommended amounts of calcium along with the proper amount of vitamin D (see below) still seems to be a case of the benefits outweighing the possible risks.

Older individuals who take in large amounts of calcium could develop a high blood calcium level, particularly if they have kidney problems, and should check with their physicians about an appropriate calcium intake.

Adequate calcium intake is important for bone health. Other benefits of taking calcium include weight reduction, lowering of the blood pressure, prevention of preeclampsia (a serious condition seen in pregnancy), prevention of colon cancer, and control of premenstrual symptoms. Different research studies come to different conclusions, so these benefits cannot be "guaranteed" until more studies become available.

People with kidney stones or who are at risk for kidney stones present a special problem when thinking about adequate calcium intake. Most kidney stones contain calcium and another chemical called "oxalate." Although taking calcium might seem like a bad idea in people with kidney stones, for most stone-formers, calcium actually reduces the risk of forming stones. This is due to the prevention of dietary oxalate (the other chemical in most stones) from getting absorbed in the intestine. However, for those people who form stones and have very high urine calcium to begin with, taking calcium without careful monitoring is a bad idea. If you are a stone-former or have family members who are, check with your doctor about how much and what kind of calcium you should take and how often your blood and urine calcium should be monitored.

Vitamin D

Why Is Vitamin D Important and How Do I Get Enough?

Vitamin D has been called the "sunshine vitamin." Even brief weekly exposure to the sun should lead to adequate amounts of vitamin D being produced in the skin and then "activated" in the liver and kidney. However, many of us spend most of our time indoors, even getting our exercise inside. We appropriately use sunscreen when going outdoors to reduce the risk of skin cancer. The same sunscreen that reduces the risk of skin cancer also interferes with the ability of our skin to make vitamin D.

Very few foods contain vitamin D. Certain fish oils, such as cod liver oil, and vitamin D-fortified products contain some vitamin D, but particularly in the case of the fortified products, it is usually not enough. Currently, it is recommended that we should take in 800 to 1,000 units of vitamin D daily. This is the amount of vitamin D contained in two quarts of milk, but few of us drink two quarts of milk daily.

The best solution is to take vitamin D supplements. There are two forms of vitamin D. Vitamin D2 comes from plants, while vitamin D3 comes from animal sources. Most reports suggest that vitamin D3 is the more active and the preferred form to take, although one report suggests that D2 may be adequate. Most calcium preparations contain vitamin D3, but this should be stated on the label. The label may be confusing in that it may talk about a serving of the vitamin/calcium supplement. A serving may be one tablet, two tablets, or more. Read the label carefully to be sure of how much calcium and vitamin D each tablet provides.

Vitamin D is essential for the proper absorption of calcium and phosphorus and for good bone health. Vitamin D is also important for proper muscle function, and people who are vitamin D deficient are fatigued and weak. Recently there has been interest in the use of large amounts of vitamin D to improve immune function and to prevent certain types of cancer. Vitamin D helps cells to reach maturity ("differentiate"), and this may be the basis of enhanced immune function and cancer prevention. However, large amounts of vitamin D in the diet can lead to complications. Vitamin D in large amounts can raise the calcium level and in some cases the phosphorus level in the blood, and raise the calcium level in the urine. Large amounts of vitamin D can also lead to bone problems. Until definitive studies are published concerning cancer prevention and immune function enhancement, people should follow their physicians' advice about just how much vitamin D to take.

Physicians can check vitamin D levels with a blood test to see if the level is adequate. Some people who consume the proper amount of vitamin D and still cannot achieve the proper level may be unable to absorb vitamin D normally. For instance, a condition known as "gluten-sensitive enteropathy" or "celiac disease" or "sprue" in which there is an abnormal response in the intestine to a certain wheat protein, is also associated with vitamin D deficiency and osteoporosis.

Rarely some diseases may cause one to have too much vitamin D in his or her bloodstream. For example, there is an inflammatory condition called "sarcoidosis," which commonly affects the lungs and can lead to vitamin D overproduction by certain immune cells. People with this condition must monitor their vitamin D and calcium intake very carefully.

Other Things to Consider

The body controls calcium levels by measuring how much calcium is in the blood and then releasing a hormone called "parathyroid hormone," or "PTH," if the calcium falls below a certain level. Parathyroid hormone activates vitamin D that comes from the diet or skin exposed to the sunlight. The active vitamin D helps absorb calcium in the intestine and mobilizes calcium from bone.

Sometimes one or more parathyroid glands (there usually are four) can become overactive regardless of the calcium level and can lead to the unnecessary activation of vitamin D and reabsorption of bone. This condition is called "hyperparathyroidism" and leads to bone damage and high calcium levels in the blood. So, a high parathyroid hormone level may be appropriate if the body is calcium and vitamin D deficient, but it is not appropriate if the body has enough vitamin D and calcium. This is an important distinction because in the case of deficiency, all that is needed is the proper amount of calcium and vitamin D. However, in the case of an overactive, dysfunctional parathyroid gland leading to high blood calcium, surgery may be required. Usually it is easy to tell the difference between an appropriate increase in parathyroid hormone due to calcium and vitamin D deficiency and the inappropriate increase in parathyroid hormone due to an abnormal parathyroid gland, which leads to a high calcium level. However, sometimes with mild disturbances it can be difficult to tell the difference, in which case an endocrinologist (a hormone and metabolic specialist) can help sort this out.

Magnesium is important for proper metabolism of calcium. Unlike calcium, magnesium is easy to absorb, readily available in many types of food, and is needed only in small amounts each day. Usually only people with bowel problems leading to malabsorption (such as chronic diarrhea), certain kidney problems, adrenal problems, or certain medications really need to take supplemental magnesium.

Finally, what about the bones? Calcium and phosphorus as well as vitamin D are essential for good bone health. But osteoporosis, the most common metabolic bone disease, is not really due to just a calcium or phosphorus deficiency. It is mostly an inherited condition in which the normal lifelong removal by the body of small amounts of old fragile bone is not matched by the proper replacement of new supple, fracture-resistant bone. However, a lack of calcium (and sometimes phosphorus) and vitamin D will increase bone loss dramatically because of the body's need to keep the blood and cellular calcium normal. This makes the osteoporosis much worse. A deficiency of calcium, vitamin D, and phosphorus will lead to a softening of the bones due to too much of the flexible bone collagen not being stiffened by the deficient, hard calcium phosphate crystal. This condition is called "osteomalacia" or "rickets" in children and is just as bad as osteoporosis, although the solution is simple: enough calcium, phosphorus, and vitamin D.

Other nutrients in addition to calcium and vitamin D are important for bone health. These include protein, copper, and vitamin K. For the most part, any condition that is associated with malnutrition or poor nutrition will be associated with some element of protein malnutrition and negative effects on the bone. Some less common medical illnesses, as well as side effects of certain drugs, are associated with problems of copper and vitamin K nutrition and can lead to osteoporosis.

Some Final Thoughts

Calcium and vitamin D deficiency are easy to prevent, but they are also easy to overlook. For many years there may be no symptoms, but then fracture, muscle weakness, and other problems related to disordered metabolism occur and, at least in the case of fracture, may cause permanent disability. Keeping calcium and vitamin D supplements in full view on the table is a good way to remember to take them. It is always best to first check with your doctor about the recommended dosing. This is one place where an old piece of advice fits well when it comes to calcium and vitamin D: an ounce of prevention really is worth a pound of cure.

Suggested Readings

AACE Power of Prevention. Endocrine Health. "Osteoporosis." http://www.powerofprevention.com/osteoporosis.php (accessed August 23, 2008).

AACE Power of Prevention, Endocrine Health. "Parathyroid." http://www.powerofprevention.com/parathyroid.php (accessed August 23, 2008).

Holick, Michael F. Vitamin D Deficiency Medical Progress. The New England Journal of Medicine. 2007; 357: 266.

Nutrition and Bone Disorders. *The Mount Sinai School of Medicine Complete Book of Nutrition.* New York: St. Martin's Press, 1990: 574.

Oregon State University Linus Pauling Institute Web site. http://lpi.oregonstate.edu/infocenter/minerals/calcium/ (accessed August 2, 2008).

Table. Food sources and calcium provided

Food	Serving	Calcium (mg)	Servings needed to equal the absorbable calcium in 8 oz of milk
Milk	8 ounces	300	1.0
Yogurt	8 ounces	300	1.0
Cheddar cheese	1.5 ounces	303	1.0
Pinto beans	1/2 cup, cooked	45	8.1
Red beans	1/2 cup, cooked	41	9.7
White beans	1/2 cup, cooked	113	3.9
Tofu, calcium set	1/2 cup	258	1.2
Bok choy	1/2 cup, cooked	79	2.3
Kale	1/2 cup, cooked	61	3.2
Chinese cabbage	1/2 cup, cooked	239	1.0
Broccoli	1/2 cup, cooked	35	4.5
Spinach	1/2 cup, cooked	115	16.3
Rhubarb	1/2 cup, cooked	174	9.5
Fruit punch with calcium citrate malate	8 ounces	300	0.62

Source: Linus Pauling Institute. http://lpi.oregonstate.edu/infocenter/minerals/calcium/ (accessed July 12, 2010).

Food Tables

Chapter 4.10

Nutrition and Chronic Diseases

Michael Via, MD

What Is Chronic Disease?

Chronic disease is defined as a disease that lasts for more than six months, though most of the time the disease lasts much longer—years or even decades. A person with a chronic disease will often live with the condition for the remainder of his or her lifetime. Adjustments to one's daily routine are often necessary to reduce suffering and optimize quality and enjoyment of life. Actually, chronic disease exists simply because modern medicine has been so successful in treating disease and preventing early deaths. Some examples of chronic disease are kidney disease (see chapter 4.4, "Nutrition and Kidney Problems"), heart disease (see chapter 4.7, "Nutrition and Heart Disease"), and cancer (see chapter 4.8, "Nutrition and Cancer").

People with chronic disease may require specific dietary restrictions. They also frequently experience decreased physical activity, appetite, food intake, and body weight. This prolonged state of negative energy balance (metabolic needs are more than dietary calories) may produce a significant amount of unintentional loss of body weight, called "wasting."

Another type of body change that occurs with chronic disease is called "cachexia." In this condition, there is a loss of muscle and organ function, with little or no loss of fat. Cachexia is caused by chronic inflammation, and there is often a change in the way protein is made in the body. Body weight can remain the same, decrease over time, or even increase. When there is weight gain, it is due to swelling (called "edema") that results from depletion of a protein called "albumin." Some examples of chronic disease that are associated with inflammation and cachexia include cancer (discussed in depth in chapter 4.8); rheumatoid arthritis; chronic obstructive pulmonary disease, which includes emphysema and chronic bronchitis; and heart failure.

Rheumatologic Disease

Rheumatologic diseases are those that affect the bones, joints, ligaments, tendons, and other soft tissues. They are often associated with problems with the immune system. Specifically, the body's own immune system attacks these tissues as part of an "autoimmune" process. Examples of rheumatologic disease include "rheumatoid arthritis" (RA), "lupus," and "scleroderma." These types of diseases progress slowly over years to decades. They can lead to debilitation and decreased physical activity, both of which severely affect a person's quality of life and longevity.

Rheumatoid arthritis causes bone and joint destruction, which results in stiffness, weakness, and difficulty with walking or performing daily tasks. The heightened degree of inflammation associated with RA may explain the cachexia that is common to this disease. Despite having a higher body mass index and increased weight, people with RA tend to have a lower muscle mass and can be truly undernourished. An adequate dietary intake of calories, proteins, and fats is therefore very important for optimal health in these people.

While it is important to encourage food intake, dietary changes that reduce inflammation may help to alleviate the symptoms of RA. Several studies have suggested that an increase in dietary omega-3 fatty acids improves symptoms of joint pain, muscle stiffness, and overall quality of life in people with RA. This can be accomplished with fish oil capsules (3 grams a day) or the "Mediterranean diet." This diet emphasizes healthy food choices that are high in unsaturated fats and incorporates fruits, vegetables, fish, olive oil, legumes, whole grains, nuts, and red wine. Other dietary modifications, such as low-fat diets, vegetarian or vegan diets, and antioxidant supplementation do not clearly benefit people with RA.

Adequate calcium and vitamin D intake is also important for bone health in people with rheumatologic disease. This is because chronic inflammation can decrease bone mineral density and increase the risk for osteoporosis. In addition, many of these people are treated with steroids, which when dosed for a long time, can directly harm the bones and diminish mobility, in addition to increasing the body fat mass and reducing the muscle mass.

Pulmonary Disease

The lungs are designed to optimize oxygen (O_2) and carbon dioxide (CO_2) exchange through a series of airways and specialized air sacs called "alveoli." There is also a rich supply of small blood vessels, called "capillaries," for the movement of these gases. Successful lung function depends on the ability to maintain open airways.

In chronic obstructive pulmonary disease (COPD), years of exposure to cigarette smoke or other environmental toxins lead to destruction of the protein structure that keeps the airways open. This makes breathing difficult because there is an impaired exchange of O_2 and CO_2. People with COPD often have lower levels of O_2 and higher levels of CO_2 in their bloodstream. Exercise, climbing stairs, or even walking can cause shortness of breath, wheezing, and coughing.

People with COPD are at particularly high risk for weight loss and wasting syndrome; about half are malnourished. This is a result of a decrease in appetite due to inflammation in the body (cachexia) and an increase in the amount of energy required for breathing. Those with an abnormally low body weight have a worse prognosis. People with COPD typically need to take in higher than usual amounts of calories to maintain their body weights. This is often best accomplished by consuming 5 to 6 smaller meals per day.

One strategy for the nutritional management of people with COPD involves reducing the carbohydrate intake. Metabolism of carbohydrates is known to produce more CO_2 than the metabolism of fats in healthy individuals. So, by lowering the carbohydrate intake, it is hoped to lower CO_2 levels in people with COPD. However, this theory was disproven by several research studies. These studies failed to show a decrease in CO_2 levels or any change in symptoms of shortness of breath or exercise tolerance. Therefore, at this point, a high-fat/low-carbohydrate diet is not recommended in COPD.

Research scientists have also investigated the use of antioxidants as potential treatment for COPD. A unique property of lung tissue is that it has direct contact with the outside environment. As mentioned, COPD results from repeated environmental insults, especially exposure to tobacco smoke. Tobacco smoke is known to cause oxidative damage by generating free radicals through many different chemical reactions. Naturally produced antioxidants can protect lung tissue from environmental damage. For example, those with COPD and higher levels of vitamin E and β-carotene in their diet can have less coughing and shortness of breath. This finding is interesting, but the exact mechanism of this relationship remains unclear. Perhaps those people with less severe COPD have a more balanced diet anyway and eat more antioxidant-rich foods than those with more severe COPD. Until more studies are done, we can only acknowledge the potential benefit of antioxidants as part of healthy eating in people with COPD, without actually recommending specific antioxidants as if they were proven treatments.

People with COPD, like those with RA, may be treated with steroids from time to time. The bad effects of steroids on the bones may be offset to some extent by adequate vitamin D and calcium intake as well as certain medications. Therefore, calcium and vitamin D supplements are usually recommended.

Heart Failure

Congestive heart failure (CHF) is a chronic condition that occurs when the heart can no longer pump the blood sufficiently to meet the demands of the body. This can result from long-standing high blood pressure or after the heart sustains damage from a heart attack. Congestive heart failure can also occur after receiving certain types of chemotherapy (such as adriamycin) with certain nutritional deficiencies (such as thiamine), or after certain viral infections. People with CHF have shortness of breath and difficulty with exercise and daily activities. Some people with CHF can walk only a short distance before stopping to catch their breath. Others with severe CHF cannot even get out of bed. Many people with CHF hold onto too much water and salt, which can cause swelling around the ankles or fluid in the lungs. Despite modern medical therapy, about half of those with CHF will die within four years after they are diagnosed with the disease.

An important feature of CHF is malnutrition, which can take the form of cachexia. About two-thirds of people with CHF have muscle wasting; although, only about 15 percent meet the criteria for "cardiac cachexia" (6 percent of body weight lost over six months). People with CHF and cachexia have approximately three times the death rate compared to those without cachexia. One research study showed that providing just 600 calories extra to people with CHF improved their weight and exercise tolerance. Extra calories in the form of calorically dense liquid supplements (so the amount of fluid is kept at a minimum) may therefore be considered in people with CHF who are not meeting their goals for caloric intake.

General Advice for People with Chronic Disease and Their Families

The best advice for those with chronic disease is to adopt dietary habits that provide an adequate amount of calories, protein, minerals, and vitamins. The goal for calorie intake is typically in the range of 25 to 35 calories per kilogram per day and protein requirements range from 0.8-1.2 grams per kilogram per day.

In the real world, this means that people with chronic disease should have frequent, balanced meals. It may be helpful to rest before eating in order to finish a meal. The largest meal of the day should be planned around times when energy levels are at their highest. Frequently, this is the first meal of the day: breakfast. It may be helpful to eat foods that are easy to chew such as mashed potatoes, fish, or other soft meats that are baked or stewed. Milkshakes or nutritional supplements like Boost, Ensure, Sustacal, or Carnation Instant Breakfast can be helpful in situations where there are not enough calories in a daily meal plan. Nutrient-dense foods such as peanut butter and jelly sandwiches can also provide a higher amount of calories.

Daily vitamin and mineral supplements are generally recommended, with an extra intake of vitamin D and calcium to combat osteoporosis, which is common to people with chronic disease. At least 1,200 international units (IU) of vitamin D and 1,000-1,200 milligrams of calcium should be taken each day, usually split into two or three doses. This is usually equivalent to taking one multivitamin and two tablets of calcium plus vitamin D supplements every day, depending on the brand of supplements (see the Nutrition Facts Label for the precise amounts). Sodium should be minimized if possible.

People with chronic disease may have difficulty with meal preparation and with food shopping due to their underlying disease. In these instances, some suggest the use of ready-made microwaveable meals. If family members are available, shopping and preparing foods that are enjoyed and actually consumed is generally more important than trying to meet specific goals. For instance, providing ice cream sundaes to elderly people can frequently result in greater food intake, with proper amounts of protein, than trying to force a standard diet of meat, starch, and vegetables.

Even though getting enough calories in the diet is important for those with chronic disease, some disease-specific modifications may be helpful, such as including increased omega-3 fatty acid intake in RA and low-sodium diet with vitamin supplementation in CHF. In situations where family members are not available, assisted living or other social programs such as Meals on Wheels may also be helpful in providing nutritional care for those with chronic disease.

Chronic disease affects many aspects of a person's life. Many of the symptoms of chronic disease and the overall prognosis may be directly related to nutritional status. Adequate dietary intake and disease-specific dietary modifications can improve symptoms and quality of life dramatically.

Suggested Reading

Centers for Disease Control and Prevention. "Physical activity and good nutrition: Essential elements to prevent chronic diseases and obesity." http://www.cdc.gov/nccdphp/publications/aag/dnpa.htm (accessed on October 25, 2008).

GreenFacts. "Scientific facts on diet and nutrition: Prevention of chronic diseases." http://www.greenfacts.org/en/diet-nutrition/ (accessed on October 25, 2008).

World Health Organization. "Diet, nutrition and the prevention of chronic diseases: report of the joint WHO/FAO expert consultation." http://www.who.int/dietphysicalactivity/publications/trs916/download/en/index.html (accessed on October 25, 2008).

Chapter 4.11

Artificial Nutrition

M. Molly McMahon, MD

"Artificial nutrition" is nutrition that is administered to a person by a feeding tube into the intestinal tract (called "enteral tube feeding") or by a catheter into the bloodstream (called "parenteral nutrition" or "intravenous nutrition"). In general, artificial nutrition is used to nourish people who are unable to eat adequate nutrition by mouth safely. While called artificial, the nutrients are not artificial. They are the same nutrients as those found in food, but in liquid form.

Eating brings us so much enjoyment, and not being able to eat can be very difficult. Yet many people who require artificial nutrition for long periods of time have active, independent lives. Medical team members want to provide enough information so that patients are not intimidated by this type of nutritional treatment.

Enteral Tube Feeding

What Is Enteral Tube Feeding?

During normal digestion, the food taken by mouth goes down the esophagus into the stomach and then into the intestines. Enteral tube feeding is a method of administering liquid nutrition products, which are called "enteral formulas," into the gastrointestinal (GI) tract through a feeding tube.

Tube feeding is used to provide nutrition to people with a functioning GI tract who are not able to eat by mouth and/or digest enough nutrition safely. Examples include patients following strokes who have difficulty swallowing or patients with a blockage (or "obstruction") of the esophagus, like from esophageal cancer. These patients can have a feeding tube placed past the obstruction into the stomach or the small bowel. Generally, tube feeding, rather than parenteral nutrition, should be used for patients with a GI tract that works normally. Tube feeding improves the health of the cells lining the GI tract, has fewer complications than parenteral nutrition, and costs less than parenteral nutrition.

Swallow Evaluation

Before determining if a tube feeding should be considered, doctors will ask the patient about his or her swallowing abilities. For instance, does it take more effort and time to move food or liquid from the mouth into the stomach? Do foods or liquids feel like they stick or become stuck?

Does the patient cough or choke while eating? Is it easier to take liquids than solids? Has the patient had repeated bouts of pneumonia? Is the patient unable to swallow anything?

If the patient seems to have trouble swallowing, a formal swallowing evaluation and test called a "videofluoroscopy" is recommended. A videofluoroscopy is a videotaped x-ray of the swallowing process. For some patients, the only safe option is to avoid eating by mouth altogether. Other patients may be permitted to eat certain textures and consistencies of food by mouth but require artificial nutrition as well. For those with swallowing problems, the swallow evaluation should be repeated periodically to see if nutrition by mouth would be safe.

Medical Nutrition Consultation

Prior to decisions being made about beginning tube feeding, the patient meets with a physician and possibly also with a registered dietitian or nurse who is experienced in the use of enteral tube feeding. The medical team reviews current nutritional intake and body weight changes, swallowing status, and swallowing study results to determine whether any intake by mouth is safe. The patient's medical prognosis and the wishes of the person regarding the use of tube feeding are also considered. The type of feeding tube and nutrition formula are then recommended.

Tube-Feeding Formula

While there are many different types of tube-feeding formulas, each one provides the correct balance of carbohydrates, fat, protein, minerals, vitamins, and water. The health-care provider who is supervising the nutrition will determine which tube-feeding formula and how much volume should be administered to meet the nutritional needs. Although there is water in the tube-feeding formula, patients will need additional fluids given through the tube to stay adequately hydrated and keep the tube from getting clogged. These additional fluids are referred to as "flushes" and may be plain water or salt water (called "saline"). An additional vitamin/mineral supplement may also be required for adequate vitamin intake, especially during periods of stress or significant illness. There are many type and brands of tube feeds, many of which are specialized according to heart, lungs, kidney, or liver function.

Short-term Feeding Tube Access

Enteral feeding devices can enter the GI tract through the nose ("nasoenteral") or through the abdominal wall surgically or "percutaneously" by using a device called an "endoscope" through the mouth, down the esophagus; placement is guided visually and then a small puncture is made through the abdominal wall to attach the tube. The end of the tube can be in the stomach ("surgical G-tube" or percutaneous endoscopic gastrostomy [PEG]; the word *gastro-* means related to the stomach) or in a part of the small bowel called the "jejunum" ("surgical J-tube" or percutaneous endoscopic jejunostomy [PEJ]). The doctor will make a recommendation whether to provide tube feeds into the stomach or jejunum based on the function of the stomach. Delivering tube feeds into the jejunum is an effective way to bypass a stomach that does not work well. Nasoenteral tube tip location should be confirmed by x-ray before the formula is administered. Here the tip location can be in the stomach ("nasogastric") or jejunum ("nasojejunal").

Long-term Feeding Tube Access

Generally, nasoenteral tubes are not used for more than a month. For long-term feeding, tubes that exit the abdominal wall often are recommended for patient comfort, to decrease the chance of accidental removal or movement of the tube, and to prevent sinus inflammation from prolonged use of a tube that enters through the nose. Long-term feeding tube access can be placed by medical specialists in digestive disorders, called "gastroenterology," who perform endoscopy. Some radiologists and surgeons can also perform endoscopic placement of feeding tubes.

Gastric (Stomach) vs. Jejunal (Small Bowel) Tube Feeding

Generally, tube feeding delivered into the stomach is preferred over tube feeding delivered into the jejunum, part of the small bowel. Formula feeding into the stomach is more similar to eating by mouth. The tube feeding formula is provided two to four times daily over forty-five to sixty minutes using a gravity flow tube feeding bag. A "residual" check is done to determine if the tube is in the proper position for feeding and to be sure the formula leaves the stomach properly. The residual is the amount of formula left in the stomach after the previous feeding. This is determined by pulling back on a large plastic syringe attached to the feeding tube to see how much tube feed is still in the stomach.

Patients who might require jejunal feeding include those with severe motility disorders of the stomach, such as "diabetic gastroparesis" (that is, the stomach does not empty contents well), or obstruction of the stomach, in which case the feeding must be provided past the obstruction. Jejunal tube feeding is provided by an infusion pump over a longer period of time. Often, the formula is administered at night while the person is sleeping. Residual checks are generally not needed with jejunal feedings.

Tube Feeding Complications

Tube feeding can cause "aspiration." Aspiration occurs when stomach contents or secretions go into the lungs, and this can result in a serious lung infection, called "aspiration pneumonia." This risk is lessened by keeping the head and chest of the person receiving tube feeding raised above the level of the stomach during the feeding and then for thirty to sixty minutes after the feeding. There always is the risk of aspirating one's own saliva with a swallowing problem, so tube feeding does not completely eliminate the risk of aspiration. For patients receiving jejunal tube feeding, the tube can move back from the small bowel into the stomach. In this case, checking the residual can be helpful.

Long-term Tube Feeding

Many people in a home setting or nursing home receive long-term tube feeding. However, since insurance coverage varies, third-party payers should be contacted for information regarding reimbursement and proper documentation.

Education is provided to the patient and family/caregiver about preparing and administering the tube feeding formula, proper amount and timing of flushes, skin and abdominal site care, and medication administration. Patients/families should know the type of tube, location of tube tip (stomach or small bowel), tube feeding formula program, how to check the residual volume (if necessary), and the nutrition formula. A home health-care company representative will assist with arranging and delivering equipment and supplies.

Health-care team members will monitor body weights and weight trends of the patient, fluid balances (for example, amounts of tube feeds, any intake by mouth, urine output, diarrhea if any), residual volume check results, feeding tolerance (presence or absence of abdominal pain and abdominal distention), diarrhea or constipation, and lab studies. Blood studies help monitor blood sugar level, electrolytes, vitamins, and minerals as determined by the medical team. Adjustments may be made to the tube feeding formula and/or the flushes based on the blood test results and overall clinical status.

Liquid drug preparations are preferred for feeding tube administration to lessen the chance of clogging the feeding tube. If a liquid form is not available, certain medicines can be crushed for administration. One should crush the medication to a fine powder and mix with water just before use. Each dose should be separately administered and a water flush administered between doses and after the last dose in order to lessen the chance of clogging the tube. Certain drugs should not be administered by tube, so one should always check with a nurse or doctor before starting a new medication through the tube.

The patient should also contact the doctor if the feeding tube becomes clogged, is removed, or if the patient develops weight change, fever, stomach pain, stomach distention, significant diarrhea or constipation, dehydration (thirst, decreased volume of urine, or dark-colored urine), and/or soreness, discharge, or redness around the site where the feeding tube exits in the abdominal wall.

Parenteral Nutrition

What Is Parenteral Nutrition?

Normal digestion and absorption of foods occurs through the GI tract. If the GI tract cannot be used because of disease, a patient may receive nutrition through the bloodstream. This is called parenteral nutrition (PN). The person may need PN for a short term during hospitalization or may require PN for months or for life. Conditions that might require PN include inflammatory bowel disease (Crohn's disease or ulcerative colitis), surgical bowel removal (short bowel syndrome), or abnormal bowel function (motility disorder where the stomach and small bowel do not empty secretions or food normally, or nutrient absorptive disorders such as damage from radiation or chemotherapy).

PN that is required at home is called "home parenteral nutrition," or HPN. Before recommending HPN, the doctor may need to complete certain tests to establish a medical need for HPN, which also is required for insurance coverage. The medical team will review the nutrition and medical history and prognosis of the medical condition, and always discuss the wish of the patient regarding HPN use.

PN Catheter

Various types of catheters are used for PN. These include central access devices, such as a Hickman catheter, a port or an implantable access device, a Groshong catheter, or a peripherally inserted central catheter called a PICC (pronounced as "pick"). A PICC is inserted in the upper arm, while the other types of central catheters are inserted in the neck or chest. Sometimes, PN is infused through an ordinary peripheral IV in the forearm. This is called "peripheral parenteral nutrition," or "PPN" (compared with "central parenteral nutrition" or "total parenteral nutrition" [TPN]). PPN can generally provide only a portion of a patient's total nutritional needs since it infuses through a smaller peripheral IV.

The nutrition specialist will recommend the most appropriate catheter for a patient. Confirming the location of the catheter and tip is needed before infusing central PN. The catheter tip should be in the superior vena cava, a large blood vessel that enters the right atrium of the heart. Catheter tip confirmation is not needed for PPN.

PN Formula

PN formulas provide fluid, calories, fat, carbohydrate, protein, electrolytes, minerals, and vitamins. Usually all of these ingredients are together in one bag that is white in color. Sometimes, the lipid (fat) part of the formula is contained in a separate bag that is white, and the other bag containing the remaining ingredients is yellow, due to the color of the vitamins. The doctor will determine appropriate nutrient amounts for a particular medical condition and will clarify nutrition goals. Some patients may eat small amounts of food in addition to receiving PN. PN is administered by an infusion pump. Changes in body weight or abnormal lab test results will require changes in the formula content.

PN and HPN Complications

Patients receiving PN may experience catheter problems, including catheter misplacement, infection, or clots. Catheter infections may lead to bloodstream infections that are serious. Treatment may require infusion of antibiotics through the central catheter to fight the infection or catheter removal until the infection has cleared followed by the placement of a new catheter.

Common metabolic complications include abnormalities of blood sugar, electrolytes, or minerals. Providing more calories than required can result in serious problems, including elevated blood sugar (that can lead to infection), abnormal liver blood tests, and breathing problems. Bone disease may also occur in a patient on HPN.

Health-care team members monitor body weight trends and blood tests for levels of blood sugar, triglycerides, vitamins, minerals, and electrolytes. The PN formula and volume are then modified as indicated.

Home Parenteral Nutrition (HPN)

HPN should be used under the direction of a physician and team skilled in this form of nutrition. This team will guide the type of catheter that is desired for PN and the education needed to prepare and administer the PN formula using a sterile technique, meaning careful handling of sterile products in a clean environment. A home health-care company will assist with arranging and delivering equipment and supplies. Patients need education in PN administration, care of the access device and equipment, PN program and infusion schedule, medication administration, and monitoring program. PN is administered by infusion pump and is often infused at night to allow freedom from the infusion pump during the day. The patient should know the type of catheter used and the specific nutrition program and infusion schedule prescribed. Regular communication is required between the patient receiving HPN and the health-care team.

Reporting HPN Problems to the Medical Team

Patients should notify their health-care providers if they develop fever, chills, or redness or discharge at the catheter exit site as this may be a sign of infection. Patients should report any problems with catheter infusion. Patients should also be told how often body weight should be checked and be given guidelines about weight change that should prompt a phone call to the medical team.

"Advanced Directives" – Letting Your Doctor Know If You Will Want Artificial Nutrition

This decision to initiate long-term tube feeding or parenteral nutrition requires clarification of the anticipated medical outcome. Long-term nutrition can help improve medical outcomes in many situations but not in others, including end-stage cancer and severe dementia.

If a patient is unable to make his or her own health-care decision, the doctor will review the advance directive, if available. An advance directive allows a patient to express future health-care goals if decision-making capacity is no longer present. In general, there are two types of advance directives: the living will and the durable power of attorney for health care. The living will allows a patient to list interventions and actions that should or should not be taken in certain situations (e.g., long-term tube feeding or PN). For instance, when and for how long would a patient want to be fed by artificial nutrition? Would it matter what the prognosis was? The durable power of attorney for health care is a legal document that designates an individual to make medical decisions on behalf of the patient in the event that he or she is unable to do so.

The issues related to serious illness or accidents are not easy to discuss, but it is easier on everyone if a patient has an advance directive in place before facing a serious illness or accident. Patients should have open discussions with the people they have designated as decision makers. This person will use the living will as a guide but will need to interpret a patient's wishes when unexpected developments are not specifically addressed by the living will.

Selected Readings

McMahon MM, Hurley DL, Kamath PS, Mueller PS. Medical and ethical aspects of long-term enteral tube feeding. Mayo Clinic Proc 2005;80(11):1461-1476.

Hammond KA, Szezycki, Pfister D. Transitioning to home and other alternate sites. In: Gottschlich MM, ed. *The Science and Practice of Nutrition Support. A Case-Based Core Curriculum.* Kendall/Hunt Publishing Company; Dubuque, IA. 2001.

Kovavevivh DS, Canada T, Lown D. Monitoring home and other alternate site nutrition support. In: Gottschlich MM, ed. *The Science and Practice of Nutrition Support. A Case-Based Core Curriculum.* Kendall/Hunt Publishing Company; Dubuque, IA. 2001.

The Oley Foundation. http://www.oley.org/ (accessed on August 2, 2008). This is a website with a lot of valuable information for patients on home infusion of total parenteral (intravenous) nutrition.

Chapter 4.12

Dietary Supplements

Jeffrey I. Mechanick, MD, FACP, FACE, FACN

These days most conversations about nutrition, whether formal with a doctor or informal with friends or family, will almost always involve "supplements." In order to have a healthy lifestyle that includes a healthy diet, the role for dietary supplements must be made clear. Certainly, different ideas exist as one searches for the correct answer to the question: "Should I be taking any supplements?" These range from "more is better" to "none, unless you have a true deficiency."

In addition, the background of the person providing the advice is important to consider. For instance, health-care practitioners who use "alternative," "complementary," "unconventional," "holistic," or any other non-traditional method will base their advice on experience, testimonial, cultural and folk practices, and other non-scientific means. If the person recommending a dietary supplement also is the person selling the dietary supplement, then "profiteering" and "quackery" on the part of that health-care practitioner is a concern. That is, the motivation for recommending the dietary supplement may be making money rather than trying to improve a person's health. On the other hand, purely "traditional" American doctors will base their decisions on what they were taught in Western-style medical schools, which is essentially based on scientific evidence. Obviously, there are many gray areas in these scenarios where there is insufficient evidence or even compelling experience.

What are dietary supplements? In 1994, Congress passed the Dietary Supplement Health and Education Act and defined dietary supplements as (1) a vitamin or mineral, (2) an herb or other plant-derived chemical, (3) an amino acid, (4) another dietary substance that increases the total dietary intake, or (5) a concentrate, metabolite, constituent, or extract of the above. Glandular extracts, like thyroid, pituitary, or adrenal extracts, are also dietary supplements and should generally be avoided. Most dietary supplements do not require a prescription. Some higher potency dietary supplements are termed "nutraceuticals." Examples of nutraceuticals are the soy chemical ipriflavone, the fish oil omega-3 fatty acid, and the combination preparations of folic acid, vitamin B12, and vitamin B6.

Meal substitutes, like Ensure® or Boost®, or whole foods, even "functional" foods, are not dietary supplements. "Medical foods" are also not dietary supplements. Medical foods are recognized by the US Food and Drug Administration as a food that is prescribed by a physician for patients who have a specific nutrient need and is labeled that way, and the patient remains under the physician's ongoing care. One example is a food formulated without the amino acid phenylalanine for patients with the disease phenylketonuria (PKU disease).

One safe way to take advantage of the availability of dietary supplements and at the same time not expose yourself to unnecessary risks is to consult your physician about any dietary supplement you are interested in taking. Many supplements interact with one another, with other medications, and with certain foods. If your physician is unable to answer your questions, then a referral to a physician with expertise in nutrition may be a good option.

If you take a supplement, look for the "USP" (United States Pharmacopeia) designation on the label. This ensures the product meets the standards for strength, purity, disintegration, and dissolution established by the USP. Remember that just because the label states a certain ingredient is present it does not mean it actually is or that it is there at the specified concentrations. It also does not mean that it actually works and is safe. Also, make sure you understand the recommended dosing that is provided on the label: do you take one or two capsules, packets, or teaspoonfuls? If you are purchasing dietary supplements, then try to purchase brand names. Lastly, avoid "megadosing," where you are ingesting far more than 100 percent of the daily value of the nutrient.

At present, AACE and the American College of Endocrinology (ACE) do not endorse or recommend the use of unproven dietary supplements mainly due to safety concerns. Just because a dietary supplement is "natural" does not mean it is necessarily better, less expensive, or even safer than a "drug." For instance, boron has been recommended by some alternative medicine practitioners to promote bone health, reduce the pain associated with arthritis, and increase testosterone and muscle mass. However, these *unproven* benefits are outweighed by the *proven* risks for acute poisoning. In conclusion, discuss the issue of dietary supplements with your doctor.

Supplement	**Benefits**	**Risks**
Calcium	bone health	excess calcium
Fiber	decreases certain cancers	rare
Folic acid	decreases certain birth defects	excess can mask B12 deficiency
Multivitamin	to prevent deficiencies in at-risk persons (pregnant, elderly, after weight-loss surgery, athletes, poor diet, and with certain	rare
Psyllium seed husk	healthy circulation	rare
Vitamin D	bone heath	excess calcium and phosphorus
Selected Dietary Supplements with Weakly Proven or Unproven Benefit and/or Safety		
Supplement	Proposed Benefits	Risks
Chromium	diabetes	rare
Coenzyme Q10	"statins"	rare
Garlic	improves circulation	rare
Ginkgo biloba	improves thinking	could cause bleeding
Magnesium	diabetes	excess magnesium
Milk thistle	helps the liver	rare
Saw palmetto	decreases prostate enlargement	rare
St. John's Wort	depression	interaction with other drugs
Vanadium	diabetes	rare

Summary of Safe Usage of Supplements

- Consult your physician on all supplements considered or taken.
- Avoid using supplements with unproven benefits and safety.
- Look for the USP designation on the label.
- Try to purchase brand names whenever possible.
- Avoid megadosing.

Selected Readings

Herbalgram. http://herbalgram.org/ (accessed on November 2, 2008).

Mechanick JI, Brett EM, Chausmer AB, et al. "AACE Medical Guidelines for the Clinical Use of Dietary Supplements and Nutraceuticals." http://www.aace.com/pub/pdf/guidelines/Nutraceuticals2003.pdf (accessed on November 2, 2008).

Phytochemical and Ethnobotanical Databases. http://www.ars-grin.gov/duke/ (accessed on November 2, 2008).

Quackwatch. http://www.quackwatch.com/ (accessed on November 2, 2008).

US National Institutes of Health Office of Alternative Medicine. http://altmed.od.nih.gov/ (accessed on November 2, 2008).

Chapter 4.13

Nutrition and the Athlete

Philip Rabito, MD, FACE, CNSP

Introduction

There are many factors that have a large impact in determining the success of an athlete. These factors include genetic endowment, training, coaching, psychological fortitude, and, of course, nutrition. Nutrition plays an integral role in the performance of an athlete regardless of level or activity, from the weekend jogger to the Olympic pentathlete. There are obvious differences in nutritional strategies depending upon the particular sport played and the level at which it is performed, but there are some basic nutritional principles that should be followed.

A key nutritional goal for the athlete is to optimize body mass and composition in order to maximize performance in that particular sport. For instance, nutritional strategies that support a thin and lean frame would benefit an endurance athlete or a gymnast, whereas a diet that promotes excess body weight and muscle mass would benefit a power athlete such as a shot-putter or a football interior lineman. It is also clear that what an athlete eats can have a major impact, not only on body composition, but also on energy availability, recovery, and overall exercise performance.

Energy

One of the most important nutritional goals for the athlete is to achieve energy balance. Energy balance is the state in which the energy input, or calories eaten, essentially matches the energy output, or calories burned, with physical activity and activities of daily living. This balance is essential for maintenance of lean body mass and for optimal athletic performance.

The caloric requirement for an athlete depends upon body size and composition, gender, type of exercise and intensity, and duration of activity. Obviously, the caloric requirement of a Tour de France cyclist, who can burn over 10,000 calories a day, will differ significantly from that of a gymnast. In general, non-athletes consume energy at a rate of about 40 kilocalories per kilogram a day based on activities of daily living. An athlete would add this number to the amount of calories burned during his or her daily training in order to optimize performance and maintain body mass. The amount of calories burned during a specific physical activity is given in the table on page 191.

However, if the athlete's goal is to lose weight, then a net negative energy balance is appropriate. It is recommended that this weight loss occur slowly with minimal, daily caloric reductions over time to avoid significant reductions in lean body mass and a decline in athletic performance. Similarly, weight gain and an increase in muscle mass can be achieved by adding fat and carbohydrate calories to the diet along with intense power training. Generally speaking, the caloric intake for an athlete should be comprised of about 60 percent carbohydrates, about 25 percent fat, and about 15 percent protein.

Fuel Sources

Carbohydrates

Carbohydrates are the primary dietary energy source used for exercise. They are necessary in the diet to maintain normal blood sugar ("blood glucose") levels during exercise and to provide a source of stored energy for endurance exercise. Stored energy from carbohydrate is in the form of "glycogen," which is primarily found in the liver and muscles. Inadequate carbohydrate intake is associated with muscle fatigue, problems with brain and nerve function, and worsening athletic performance. In general, 5 to 7 grams of carbohydrate per kilogram of body weight is recommended for the average athlete and 7 to 10 grams per kilogram for the endurance athlete.

Carbohydrates in the form of starch and fiber, such as pastas, breads, cereals, and whole grains, are recommended in the daily diet. However, simple sugars, such as those found in sports drinks and gels are recommended during exercise lasting over an hour in duration, as these are more easily absorbed and less likely to cause abdominal cramping with exertion.

Carbohydrates should also be ingested within thirty minutes of completing exercise, as this technique has been shown to be the best way to replenish glycogen stores. Glycogen is the preferred fuel for the next training session or competition. It is recommended that 1.5 grams of carbohydrate per kilogram of body weight be ingested within thirty minutes of exercise, and then this should repeat in two hours for maximal carbohydrate loading.

Protein

Protein is important in the diet of an athlete mainly to help repair tissue damage incurred by exercise and to allow for an increase in body muscle. In general, athletes need more protein than non-athletes. Non-athletes require 0.8 milligrams per kilogram of body weight of protein per day, whereas endurance athletes require at least 1.2 milligrams per kilogram per day. Power athletes who are trying to increase muscle mass significantly benefit most with 1.6 milligrams per kilogram per day of protein. Protein intake greater than this has not been shown to be beneficial.

Protein should come from a variety of sources including lean meats, legumes, eggs, and dairy products. Protein supplements such as whey-based drinks can be helpful for the athlete not meeting the recommended daily protein intake, but have been associated with arrhythmias and poor outcomes when they are used in low-calorie diets as meal replacements. Specific amino acids, the building blocks for proteins, such as branched chain amino acids, have not been proven to be more effective than whole-protein supplements.

Fats

Fats are essential in the diet of the athlete mainly as an alternate source of fuel to carbohydrates. This is particularly true for prolonged, medium-intensity aerobic exercise. It is recommended that no more than 25 percent of the total caloric intake comes from fat. The best sources of fat are unsaturated fats that are liquid at room temperature, such as canola, olive, and fish oils. A diet high in saturated fats, primarily from animal meats, is not recommended, as saturated fats are associated with heart disease. During and just before exercise, fats should be avoided since they may cause abdominal discomfort and slow stomach emptying. This may adversely affect athletic performance.

Dietary Supplements

"Ergogenic" aids are dietary products that may improve athletic performance. Dietary supplements are part of a multibillion-dollar-a-year business that caters to the athlete looking for a competitive edge. Frequently, claims made by the manufacturer regarding performance enhancement are unsubstantiated in the medical literature. There have also been dietary supplements that have been associated with deaths, such as "ephedra."

In general, any dietary supplement that you may be interested in taking should be discussed with your doctor. Many dietary supplements interact with medications, foods, and even other dietary supplements in ways that can make you sick. Also, even if a dietary supplement is considered safe and your doctor does not raise any objections to its use, there are still some concerns. Specifically, the brand you purchase may not contain the labeled amount of the dietary supplement. In addition, it may contain other substances, not on the label, which can harm you. Staying healthy with healthy eating and plenty of physical activity is best done without dietary supplements (see chapter 4.12, "Dietary Supplements").

Hydration

Exercise capacity is maximized when athletes maintain proper fluid balance. Dehydration not only compromises performance, but may also put the athlete at risk for heat stroke and cardiovascular collapse in extreme conditions. Athletes can reduce the higher core body temperatures induced by physical activity by producing sweat at rates that are influenced by ambient temperatures, humidity, body size, and intensity of exercise. Body water is lost in sweat. Therefore, to stay adequately hydrated, athletes should start by pre-hydrating, or drinking before the exercise session begins. The recommendations are to have 400 to 600 milliliters (1 ½–2 ½ cups) of water three hours before the event. During the activity, the athlete should attempt to drink enough fluid so as to maintain fluid balance. This can usually be accomplished by drinking approximately ¾ to 1½ cup of fluid every fifteen minutes of exercise. Obviously, this will vary according to the conditions.

Salt, or sodium, is also lost in sweat during exercise. In extreme conditions, life-threatening "hyponatremia" (low sodium levels in the bloodstream) may develop if this salt lost in the sweat is not replaced. Salt can be taken in tablet form at approximately ½ to 1 gram every hour in events lasting more than one hour. Alternatively, for exercise lasting over one hour, sports drinks containing sugar can be used as they contain not only fluid but also energy and salt. The carbohydrate content of the drink should not exceed 8 percent as this may cause abdominal discomfort during the activity.

Cramping is a common problem particularly with endurance athletes. Although scientific evidence is lacking for the specific cause, it is recommended that the athlete stay hydrated and replenish electrolytes using sports drinks during lengthy exercise to minimize cramping.

Activity	130 pound	155 pound	190 pounds
Aerobics	354	422	518
Backpacking	413	493	604
Basketball	354	422	518
Bicycling (leisure)	236	281	345
Bicycling (racing)	944	1126	1380
Bowling	177	211	259
Catch (football or baseball)	148	176	216
Circuit training	472	563	690
Dancing	266	317	388
Golf	236	281	345
Hiking	354	422	518
Ice skating	413	493	604
Jogging	413	493	604
Pushups/Situps	266	317	388
Rowing, stationary (moderate)	502	598	733
Running (10-minute mile pace)	590	704	863
Running (7-minute mile pace)	826	985	1208
Skiing, cross-country (moderate)	472	563	690
Skiing, downhill (moderate)	354	422	518
Skiing, water	354	422	518
Snorkeling	295	352	431
Soccer, casual	413	493	604
Swimming, freestyle (moderate)	472	563	690
Tennis	413	493	604
Volleyball, noncompetitive	177	211	259
Walking (moderate)	207	246	302
Weight-lifting (moderate)	177	211	259

Table I. Calories burned during one hour of various physical activities based on different body weights (adapted from www.nutristrategy.com/activitylist.htm)

Suggested Readings

Brown University. "Health education: Sports nutrition." http://www.brown.edu/Student_Services/Health_Services/Health_Education/nutrition/sportsnut.htm (accessed on October 25, 2008).

NutriStrategy. "Calories burned during exercise." www.nutristrategy.com/activitylist.htm (accessed on October 25, 2008).

Nutrition and Well-being A to Z. "Sports nutrition." http://www.faqs.org/nutrition/Smi-Z/Sports-Nutrition.html (accessed on October 25, 2008).

Ryan, M. *Sports Nutrition for Endurance Athletes*, 2nd Edition. VeloPress, Boulder, CO, 2007.

United States Department of Agriculture. "Food and nutrition information center, lifecycle nutrition: Fitness and sports nutrition." http://fnic.nal.usda.gov/nal_display/index.php?info_center=4&tax_level=2&tax_subject=257&topic_id=1358 (accessed on October 25, 2008).

Chapter 4.14

Food Allergies and Lactose Intolerance

Himani Chandra, MD

Description of Food Allergies

A food allergy is a type of immune reaction against a protein in food. "Food allergy" is distinguished from "food intolerance," which is not immune-mediated and is often the result of a missing enzyme, such as lactase. True food allergies are classified into two broad categories: immunoglobulin E (IgE)-mediated and non-IgE-mediated.

IgE is a type of antibody, which is a protein that is part of our immune system. Antibodies attack "foreign" chemicals that could be dangerous to our bodies. Over 90 percent of food allergies are IgE-mediated. Here, IgE antibodies that are located on the surface of a certain type of immune cell, called a mast cell, bind to the food protein causing the problem. This causes the release of very strong chemicals, such as histamine. The release of histamine then leads to tissue inflammation and swelling within minutes of exposure, similar to what is seen with a bee sting but occurring in various parts of the body and not just the skin.

Non-IgE-mediated reactions, on the other hand, are mediated by a type of white blood cell called T-cells. These reactions are usually less severe and more delayed in onset, occurring hours to days after exposure. These reactions also primarily affect the cells lining the intestine and can be difficult to diagnose. The most common dietary protein associated with non-IgE-mediated reactions are due to cow's milk and soy protein found in infant formulas. Some allergies, however, do not fall into either category and are known as "mixed IgE and cell mediated disorders" because they demonstrate a combination of both mechanisms.

Prevalence of Food Allergies

Food allergies are far more common in children than in adults. In general, their prevalence rate has been increasing over the past few years. Approximately 6 to 8 percent of children less than three years of age have them as compared to 3 to 4 percent of adults. The difference in prevalence rates between children and adults is due to the fact that most children outgrow their allergies over time.

The majority of allergies arise from a short list of foods. The most common causes in infants are cows' milk and soy. Cows' milk continues to be the number one allergen in preschool-aged children, with egg coming in a close second, whereas peanuts top the list in older kids between the ages of five and eighteen years. Fish, shellfish, tree nuts, and peanuts are the four most common allergies seen in adults and also account for the most fatal reactions.

The incidence of food allergy is also culturally dependent and varies across the globe depending on the diet of the local population. The more a food is consumed in a country, the higher the incidence of allergy to it. For example, fish allergy predominates in Scandinavia, whereas rice allergy is a significant problem in Japan. On the other hand, even though the Chinese consume the same amount of peanuts as Americans, there is virtually no peanut allergy in China. This is largely due to the difference in the way the peanuts are prepared in dishes; the Chinese generally eat their peanuts boiled or fried, while Americans dry roast theirs. The higher heat involved in the dry roasting process actually makes the peanuts more likely to cause allergies by increasing their "allergic potential."

Symptoms

Whereas non-IgE-mediated reactions usually present with isolated gastrointestinal symptoms, true IgE-mediated reactions can affect nearly every body system. Classically, patients develop intensely itchy, raised, red skin welts, otherwise known as "hives" or "urticaria." Other common symptoms include swelling of the face and neck ("angioedema"), sweating, flushing, tearing, sneezing, cough, nasal congestion or runny discharge, dizziness, nausea, vomiting, diarrhea, and abdominal cramping/bloating. Severe allergic reactions can result in a life-threatening condition called "anaphylaxis," in which there is a collapse of both the cardiovascular and respiratory systems. In these cases, patients may develop a sense of choking, wheezing, extreme difficulty in breathing, dramatic drop in blood pressure, severely irregular heartbeat ("arrhythmia"), and even death if proper therapy is not administered very quickly.

Another interesting phenomenon that some people experience is known as the "oral allergy syndrome" or the "pollen-food allergy syndrome." Usually these people also suffer from pollen allergies and develop swelling and itchiness of the mouth and throat while eating certain uncooked fruits and vegetables such as apples, melons, tomatoes, celery, and cherries. The symptoms are limited to the throat in over 90 percent of people. This reaction ends within minutes when the person stops eating the particular food. The allergy-inducing proteins in the foods are killed with heat, so these people are able to eat cooked versions of the particular foods without any problems.

Around 40 percent of children with moderate to severe eczema, a skin rash also known as "atopic dermatitis," have food allergies. In these children, the skin rash gets worse with the food allergy. These children can also have other conditions like asthma and inflamed nasal passages ("allergic rhinitis"), which can both be worsened by eating particular foods as well.

Food-associated exercise-induced anaphylaxis is a fascinating but frightening allergic reaction most commonly seen in adult female athletes under the age of thirty. In this condition, patients develop itching, urticaria, angioedema, and upper airway obstruction with bronchospasm during strenuous exercise two to four hours after eating particular foods, most commonly wheat and shellfish. It is important to emphasize that these patients have absolutely no reaction to the foods if they remain at rest. The allergy only occurs with exercise.

Diagnosis of Food Allergies

In order to diagnose a true food allergy, the doctor will take a detailed clinical history, which focuses on certain foods, allergic reactions, the timing of those reactions, the response to treatments, the presence of other conditions like eczema or asthma, and a very complete family history. An "elimination diet" may then be recommended, in which one or more highly suspicious foods are totally eliminated from the diet to see if the symptoms completely resolve. In IgE-mediated disorders, usually two weeks is enough to see a good response. However, in non-IgE-mediated disorders, a good response may take up to three months to occur. If the symptoms do disappear with an elimination diet, then further testing can be obtained to clarify the exact type of food allergy that is occurring.

In suspected IgE-mediated allergies, prick/puncture skin testing can be used by allergists to make a diagnosis. A small amount of a food chemical ("allergen") is placed on the patient's bare forearm, alongside a drop of salt water ("saline") and a drop of the chemical histamine. Then a small needle is used to prick through all three areas and introduce them into the top layer of the skin. The histamine is the "positive control" to make sure the person is capable of having an allergic reaction appearing as skin swelling and redness. This is known as a wheal and flare. The salt solution is the "negative control" to make sure the person does not have a reaction that looks like an allergic reaction just because the skin is pricked. Then, if the patient is truly allergic to the food allergen pricked into the skin, there will be a typical wheal and flare. This is due to food-specific IgE antibodies located on mast cells. These antibodies attach to the food allergen and cause a sudden release of histamine from the mast cells. A wheal that is at least 3 millimeters in diameter is a positive test. This test is relatively inexpensive, not uncomfortable, and produces quick results in about fifteen minutes. Even though this test is generally safe, it must be performed in a doctor's office by a qualified expert and with the correct monitoring equipment due to the rare occasion that a true anaphylactic or life-threatening reaction occurs.

Another type of allergy test is called the "radioallergosorbent," or "RAST," test. This test is used to identify food-specific IgE antibodies in the blood without actually risking an allergic reaction. Higher concentrations of antibodies will increase the likelihood of having an allergy, but the results are not always correct. RAST tests are more expensive, not immediately available, and considered less accurate than skin testing. However, they are still better for certain patients who have had a history of a severe food-associated anaphylactic reaction in which skin testing may carry too high of a risk. Similarly, patients taking antihistamines and other medications that can mess up skin testing results, as well as those with skin diseases like severe eczema that can confuse the interpretation of skin testing, may benefit from RAST testing.

Unfortunately, there is no adequate test for suspected non-IgE-mediated food allergies. In this case, a food challenge should be performed after a trial elimination diet. This involves slowly reintroducing the food suspected of causing the allergy. If the symptoms recur, then a direct relationship between the food and the allergic response is much more likely. Again, it is crucial that this type of test be performed in a monitored medical setting, with proper equipment and medications that are readily accessible, in case the patient develops a severe life-threatening allergic reaction.

Treatment of Food Allergies

The best treatment for food allergy is to avoid the culprit food completely. Unfortunately, this is easier said than done. For one thing, many foods contain trace amounts of allergens that are not clearly labeled or identified but can be enough to trigger a significant allergic reaction. Therefore, one must be extremely vigilant in the case of small children. Steps should be taken to make sure they avoid sharing food at school lunches, eating store-bought baked goods at parties, and using crafts containing unknown substances in art class. With severe allergies, even having foods prepared on grills or skillets exposed to potential allergens can lead to contamination and an unexpected allergic reaction.

Drugs, such as antihistamines and steroids, can provide relief from symptoms, but adrenaline, or "epinephrine," is the treatment for true anaphylaxis. Those people who have a history of severe reactions should carry working epinephrine autoinjector pens at all times and know how to use them. Family members or roommates should also know how to work these epinephrine pens. In the case of small children, the staff at day-care facilities, schools, and summer camps should all be educated on the pen's proper and timely use because any delay in epinephrine administration can result in death.

Unfortunately, there is no fail-safe method to prevent the development of food allergies, but studies have shown that exclusively breast-feeding infants for the first three to six months of life lowers the risk substantially. In addition, the American Academy of Pediatrics also recommends that lactating mothers avoid peanuts and nuts, that solid foods be introduced to infants after six months of age, and that peanuts, nuts, and seafood be introduced only to children older than three.

Monitoring of People with Food Allergies

It is very important that a child with a food allergy be monitored by both a pediatrician and an allergist to assess normal growth and development, proper medication use, and current allergic status. Measures should be taken by patients, family members, and friends alike to avoid all exposures to the offending agent and to ensure that reactions are recognized and treated in a timely fashion. In patients with a history of severe anaphylactic reactions, self-injectable epinephrine pens should be checked periodically to make sure they are current, functional, and available in all settings.

Since many allergies, especially those to milk, soy, and eggs, are outgrown over time, the allergist should reevaluate children with a periodic interview and examination, RAST, and/or skin prick testing at least annually to determine if the allergy has resolved. It is important, however, to keep in mind that negative tests are not a guarantee that the allergy has completely resolved. If objective tests are negative, a supervised food challenge should be undertaken in which the culprit food is reintroduced to see if a reaction can be induced before the food is permanently integrated into the diet. With the exception of peanut allergies, once a food allergy has been shown to have definitively resolved, it rarely recurs, and consequently, there is no further need for periodic monitoring of the patient.

Lactose Intolerance

Lactose intolerance is often mistaken for milk allergy but is not an immune-mediated reaction. It is far more common than food allergies, affecting 30 to 50 million Americans and at least one out of ten people in the world. In this condition, the body does not have enough lactase enzyme in the lining of the gut to break down lactose, the main sugar found in milk and milk products. Instead of being digested properly, the lactose is formed into gas by gut bacteria, and as a result, the affected individual experiences abdominal bloating, cramping, nausea, and/or diarrhea soon after consuming dairy products.

There are three tests available to confirm a diagnosis of lactose intolerance: lactose tolerance test, hydrogen breath test, and stool acidity test. Oftentimes, the first recommendation is to avoid all lactose in the diet to see if symptoms resolve. Once diagnosed, it is a condition that can be easily treated. Infants and toddlers should avoid all lactose in their diet and have an alternative source of adequate dietary calcium and vitamin D intake. On the other hand, the majority of older children and adults can tolerate small amounts of lactose and should be encouraged to eat tiny portions of certain lactose-rich foods in order to build up their tolerance even further. For those individuals unable to endure even tiny amounts of dairy, lactose-reduced milk products and lactase enzyme tablets are readily available in supermarkets and drug stores to help with digestion and minimize symptoms.

Lactose intolerance is either inherited by a gene from both parents or acquired due to injury to the small intestine from gastrointestinal conditions like celiac disease or Crohn's disease. Its prevalence varies according to race and geography. Scandinavians have the lowest rates of lactose intolerance in the world at 3 to 8 percent, whereas nearly 100 percent of Southeast Asians suffer from lactase deficiency. Two interesting evolutionary theories have been proposed to explain this discrepancy among the world's population. Not to have the lactase enzyme was "normal" in ancient times when hunting and meat-eating were the mainstays of civilization. With the development of agriculture and a dairying tradition, adults gained a selective advantage if they developed a mutation that allowed them to have enough lactase to digest milk in times of drought or food shortage. Similarly, in countries with cold, cloudy climates in which sunlight exposure is limited, like those of Scandinavia and Northern Europe, the body's ability to produce vitamin D and absorb calcium from the diet is also severely limited. Those people with a mutation that enabled them to have a functioning lactase enzyme were able to digest milk, a rich source of calcium, and thereby have a selective advantage over their counterparts who were dying of various skeletal deformities like hip fractures. Thus, not to have lactose intolerance became protective in nature, and the mutation passed on from generation to generation until it became the dominant form of inheritance.

Suggested Resources

The Food Allergy & Anaphylaxis Network. www.foodallergy.org (accessed on August 31, 2008).

American Academy of Allergy. "Asthma, & Immunology." http://www.aaaai.org/patients/gallery/foodallergy.asp (accessed on August 31, 2008).

National Institutes of Allergy and Infectious Disease. "Food Allergy." http://www3.niaid.nih.gov/topics/foodAllergy/default.htm (accessed on August 31, 2008).

The Mayo Clinic. "Food Allergy." www.mayoclinic.com/health/food-allergy/DS00082 (accessed on August 31, 2008).

Kids With Food Allergies. www.kidswithfoodallergies.org (accessed on August 31, 2008).

Chapter 5.1

The Biochemistry of Nutrition

Michael Via, MD

While chemistry is the science of change, biochemistry focuses on change within living organisms. Biochemical reactions tightly control the basic processes of life: "homeostasis" (or the resistance to change), balance between energy supply and demand, communication among cells and cell parts, DNA function in growth and reproduction, responses to various diseases, and adaptation to changes in the environment. To this end, biochemical reactions are controlled by certain proteins known as enzymes. An adequate nutritional intake provides sufficient calories to maintain a favorable energy balance, as well as sufficient protein, vitamins, and minerals for use in metabolism and homeostasis.

Carbohydrates

Carbohydrates make up approximately 40 to 60 percent of the calories in most Western diets. Chemically, they are composed of a carbon structure that is strongly bound to oxygen and hydrogen atoms ("covalent binding"). "Monosaccharides" are simple sugars. These are composed of 3 to 7 carbon atoms with oxygen and hydrogen atoms arranged around this carbon skeleton. Monosaccharides, such as glucose, can be assembled into large molecules where the glucoses link up to form starches and dietary fiber. These larger molecules are known collectively as "polysaccharides."

Glucose, a 6-carbon simple sugar, is the most important monosaccharide in carbohydrate metabolism. It is a universal source of energy and contributes to the synthesis of a large number of biologically important molecules such as amino acids (the building blocks for protein), nucleotides (the building blocks for DNA), fatty acids (the building blocks for fat), and coenzymes (molecules that assist with chemical reactions). Plant starches are composed only of glucose and, therefore, when they are broken down by enzymes, glucose is formed. Other types of monosaccharides resulting from the breakdown of polysaccharides can be converted into glucose. Thus, the metabolism of dietary carbohydrate funnels through many pathways and eventually leads to glucose.

As an energy source, glucose is metabolized in the cell by chemical reactions that use oxygen (oxidation) and produce a high-energy chemical bond—a phosphate bond. This bond is found in the chemical adenosine tri-phosphate (ATP), which can store energy in this high-energy bond for later use. In fact, ATP is the *currency* for cellular energy. This entire process is called "oxidative phosphorylation," and it occurs in a stepwise fashion that minimizes energy lost as heat.

The first phase of glucose metabolism is termed "glycolysis" (see figure, page 205). It is a basic pathway that occurs in nearly all cells. In this process, one 6-carbon glucose molecule is broken down in several steps into two 3-carbon molecules, which are called "pyruvate." The first step of glycolysis occurs almost immediately as glucose enters the cell. On entry, a phosphorus-containing molecule is added onto the sixth glucose carbon to form the chemical glucose-6-phosphate (G6P), a process known as "phosphorylation." G6P is then converted into fructose-6-phosphate, which is, in turn, phosphorylated on the first carbon, to form fructose-1,6-diphosphate. This is the "rate-limiting," or most important, step of glycolysis, and the enzyme that catalyzes this reaction, "phosphofructokinase," is tightly regulated and sensitive to the energy needs of the cell. If ATP levels are low, or if the cell is stimulated from the outside by certain hormones, then phosphofructokinase pushes glycolysis forward. At this point, the 6-carbon skeleton of fructose-1,6-diphosphate is split into two 3-carbon sugars that are eventually converted into pyruvate.

There is a net gain of two ATP molecules formed for each glucose metabolized in the ten steps of glycolysis. In addition, there are two nicotinamide adenine dinucleotide (NADH) molecules that are formed, which will also be used for ATP synthesis in oxidative phosphorylation. The relatively small amount of energy obtained with glycolysis alone is quite sufficient for cells like bacteria. However, the complex functions of most human cells demand more energy, so additional metabolic pathways have evolved to further metabolize pyruvate and generate even more energy—the "Krebs cycle."

The second phase of glucose metabolism is the Krebs cycle (see figure, page 193), which functions within the mitochondria. These small structures inside cells are responsible for energy generation. First, the 3-carbon chemical pyruvate is converted into the 2-carbon chemical "acetyl-CoA" by the enzyme pyruvate dehydrogenase (PDH). This releases one carbon as carbon dioxide (CO_2). The 2-carbon acetyl group of acetyl-CoA is then combined with a 4-carbon sugar called "oxaloaceate" in order to form the chemical "citrate." In eight more steps, citrate is then converted back into oxaloacetate producing two CO_2 molecules, one GTP (similar to ATP) molecule, three NADH molecules, and one $FADH_2$ molecule.

The third phase of glucose metabolism is the "electronic transport chain," which also resides in the mitochondria (see figure, page 193). Here, the NADH and $FADH_2$ molecules formed in the Krebs cycle and the NADH molecule formed with glycolysis are used in a five-step oxidative phosphorylation pathway that requires oxygen and efficiently yields ATP molecules. An additional thirty-two ATPs are formed by this pathway for each molecule of glucose. This system of extracting a relatively large amount of energy in the form of ATP from glucose has allowed multicellular organisms to diversify with evolution and humans to thrive in nature.

Other biochemical pathways metabolize glucose. For example, just after a meal, when glucose is abundant, liver and muscle cells take up glucose in response to the hormone insulin. This glucose is also phosphorylated to G6P, but instead of continuing down the glycolysis pathway, the G6P molecules are assembled together to form glycogen, the storage form of carbohydrates in humans. About 6 percent of liver and 1 percent of muscle mass is glycogen, which can be converted back into glucose during periods of fasting. Depending on the metabolic needs, glycogen stores can last roughly eighteen to twenty-four hours. In the extreme setting, marathon runners and other endurance athletes can almost completely deplete their glycogen stores during athletic competition, a phenomenon known as "hitting the wall." This usually occurs around mile twenty of a marathon.

During a fast, glucose can also be synthesized from other chemicals, such as glycerol, lactate, propionate, and most amino acids (except lysine and leucine). This process is termed "gluconeogenesis." It helps maintain blood glucose levels in the normal range and provides energy for vital organs such as the kidney, brain, and heart during periods of fasting.

Glucose, a 6-carbon sugar, can also be entered into the "pentose-phosphate shunt," a pathway in which glucose is converted into ribose, a 5-carbon sugar used in RNA and DNA synthesis. Another product of this pathway is NADPH, which is also an important molecule for the prevention of oxidative damage to the cell. Glucose metabolism is the best example of how dietary carbohydrates are used in the body. Three main metabolic outcomes of glucose are given in figure 4.

Fats

Fats, which are also known as "lipids," make up 30 to 40 percent of the calories in a Western diet. Approximately 98 percent of the consumed fats are in the form of triglycerides. The rest consists of phospholipids and cholesterol. For digestion and absorption of fats, triglycerides and phospholipids are broken down into their basic components: fatty acids and a monoglyceride backbone. Several enzymes called lipases perform this reaction, the most important of which is pancreatic lipase. Lipid compounds are not water soluble, just as oil and water do not mix. Within the small intestine, bile is required to form small particles that allow fatty acids and monoglycerides to be absorbed into the bloodstream. Approximately 95 percent of ingested fats are absorbed.

After absorption, the monoglycerides and free fatty acids are put back together into triglycerides, which, along with cholesterol, are packaged with various proteins into small transport particles called chylomicrons (CM). CMs are members of a class of particles known as lipoproteins. CMs transport dietary lipids in the bloodstream to peripheral tissues and liver cells for use as an energy source or for storage. Triglycerides and cholesterol can also be synthesized in the liver from carbohydrates. This process involves diverting acetyl-CoA away from the Krebs cycle into triglycerides or cholesterol production.

In between meals, the liver cells repackage triglycerides and cholesterol into very low density lipoprotein (VLDL) particles for transport to peripheral tissues. As triglycerides are consumed from the VLDL particles by muscle cells and fat cells, the VLDLs are transformed into low density lipoprotein (LDL) particles, which contain high amounts of cholesterol. LDLs are taken up by liver cells and by fat cells. If LDL levels are high, certain cells of the immune system consume LDL particles and form fatty deposits in artery walls leading to "hardening of the arteries" or "atherosclerosis." The main cause of heart attack, stroke, and peripheral vascular disease is the buildup of these fatty deposits and the inflammation that follows. Fat cells also manufacture high density lipoprotein (HDL) particles, which transport cholesterol back to the liver for metabolism. Thus, when LDL and VLDL particles are low in number and HDL particles are plentiful, a favorable state exists that is associated with the prevention of cardiovascular disease.

Fatty acids that are derived from triglycerides are an efficient source of energy. Through the biochemical process of β-oxidation that occurs in mitochondria, 2-carbon acetyl groups are removed from fatty acids in the form of acetyl-CoA. Acetyl-CoA then enters into the Krebs cycle for eventual ATP synthesis. In the liver, three acetyl-CoA molecules can be combined to form keto-acids, or "ketone bodies." These are transported to peripheral tissues for use as a very efficient energy source, especially during periods of starvation.

β-oxidation is regulated by two hormones: insulin and glucagon. After a meal, circulating glucose is abundant, and elevated insulin levels inhibit the β-oxidation of fatty acids. On the other hand, during periods of fasting, elevated glucagon levels promote the β-oxidation of fatty acids in order to liberate energy stores, as ketone bodies, from the liver.

In addition to their use as an energy source, fats play an important role forming the "lipid bilayer" structure of cell membranes. Certain fats, particularly the polyunsaturated fatty acids, can be processed to form 20-carbon signaling molecules, which are called eicosanoids, prostaglandins, leukotrienes, hydroxy-fatty acids, and lipoxins. Two of the polyunsaturated fatty acids—linoleic, an omega-6 fatty acid, and α-linolenic, an omega-3 fatty acid—are essential in the diet since they cannot be made by the body. They have important roles in the formation of eicosanoids. Since eicosanoids are used in inflammation, achieving a proper balance of omega-3 and omega-6 fatty acids in the diet can be beneficial in preventing or treating many diseases that involve inflammation.

Proteins and Amino Acids

Proteins have many biological roles. They can be structural, such as "tubulin" or "collagen." They can function as signaling molecules, such as "insulin" or "growth hormone." They can be made into antibodies to fight disease. They can serve to carry substances through the bloodstream, such as "retinol binding protein" and "thyroid binding globulin," or they can function as enzymes for biochemical reactions. The basic structure of proteins is a chain of amino acids that is linked by peptide bonds. This chain can be folded in many different ways to form unique three-dimensional structures. The final structure of the protein will determine how it interacts with other molecules in the body.

Proteins are constantly broken down into amino acids and then reassembled to maintain their integrity. Amino acids are recycled as needed by the cell. However, since there is no long-term storage form of protein, amino acids must be consumed in the diet to meet the constant need for protein synthesis and to make up for the natural losses of nitrogen in the urine and stool.

Twelve of the twenty amino acids used in proteins can be synthesized by humans and are considered as "non-essential." "Alanine" is made from pyruvate, the end product of glycolysis. "Serine" is made from 3-phosphoglycerol, an intermediate formed during glycolysis. "Glutamine," "glutamic acid," "asparagines," and "aspartic acid" are made from intermediates of the Krebs cycle. "Histidine" is synthesized from ribose. The remaining five non-essential amino acids: glycine, proline, tyrosine, cysteine, and arginine are formed from other amino acids. In certain conditions, such as in growth or disease, histidine and arginine can become essential in the diet as their rate of endogenous production does meet their metabolic usage. They are considered "conditionally essential."

The other eight amino acids—leucine, lysine, isoleucine, valine, tryptophan, threonine, methionine, and phenylalanine—are "essential" since they cannot be sufficiently synthesized from other amino acids in humans. Furthermore, all eight must be consumed in the diet since there are no protein or amino acid stores to make up for deficiencies.

If too much of a single amino acid is consumed, or if the carbon skeleton of an amino acid is used in a separate synthetic pathway such as gluconeogenesis, a process of "deamination" takes place. In this biochemical process, amine groups are removed from amino acids by "transaminase" and "glutamate dehydrogenase" enzymes. This forms ammonium (NH_4^+) ions and aspartic acid. These intermediates enter a five-step cycle in liver cells that leads to the production of urea, a compound containing two amine groups for the efficient elimination of nitrogen. Urea is then excreted in the urine. Thus, the measure of urine urea nitrogen can be used to estimate the rate of amino acid metabolism, gluconeogenesis, and a person's protein requirements, or "nitrogen balance."

Vitamins and Minerals

Vitamins and minerals play important biological roles. They provide unique biochemical properties that are very important for enzymes to work correctly. They also demonstrate great strength as structural materials and can serve as signaling substances for cellular communication. The biological properties of vitamins and minerals (see table, page 194) are provided as a brief glimpse of their distinctive biochemical activities.

Conclusion

The macronutrients and micronutrients that comprise our diet are metabolized through a series of complex biochemical reactions. These allow humans to perform and respond properly in their environment. An understanding of these pathways can complement the knowledge of nutrition provided in this book for a more complete picture of nutritional science.

One important take-home message: These complex biochemical processes have evolved in an environment of scarce food supply and high metabolic demands (running from predators and hunting-gathering food). This biochemistry protected our ancestors from the bad effects of starvation and famine. However, we did not evolve a mechanism to protect us from too much food and too little activity. Our bodies have a very difficult time metabolizing and storing excess energy. We, therefore, become overweight and obese with overeating. We then suffer the consequences of overeating, such as insulin resistance, diabetes, hypertension (high blood pressure), heart disease, stroke, and eventually premature death. This underscores the necessity for eating in a manner that resonates with our human evolution, a manner of eating we call "healthy eating."

Selected Reading

Kinney, John M., Jeejeebhoy, K.N., Hill, Graham L., Owen, Oliver E. *Nutrition and Metabolism in Patient Care.* Philadelphia: WB Saunders Company 1998.

Lehninger, Albert L.(1993) *Principles of Biochemistry*, 2nd Ed. New York: Worth Publishers.

Machlin, Lawrence J. (1991) *Handbook of Vitamins*, 2nd Ed. New York: Marcel Dekker, INC.

Shils, Maurice. (2005) *Modern Nutrition in Health and Disease*, 10th Ed. New York: Lippincott, Williams & Williams.

Stryer, Lubert. (1995) Biochemistry, 4th Ed. New York: WH Freeman and Company.

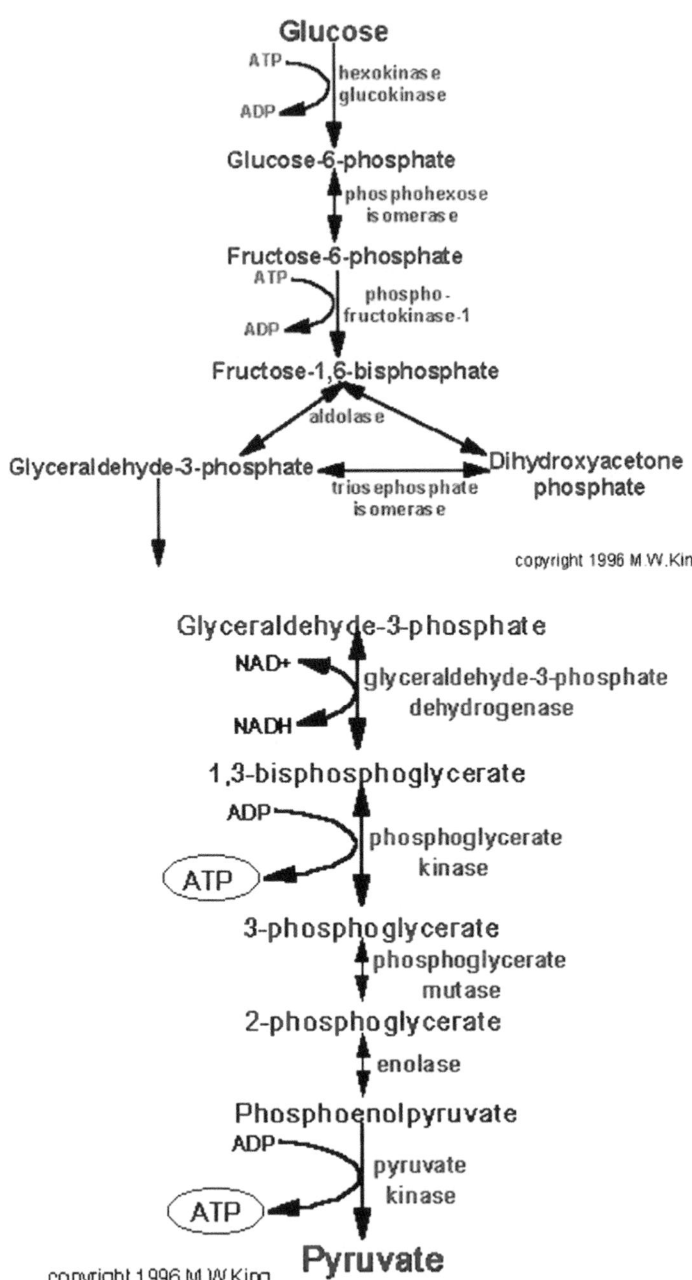

Glycolysis. (from http://www.med.unibs.it/~marchesi/glycolys.html; accessed on October 25, 2008)

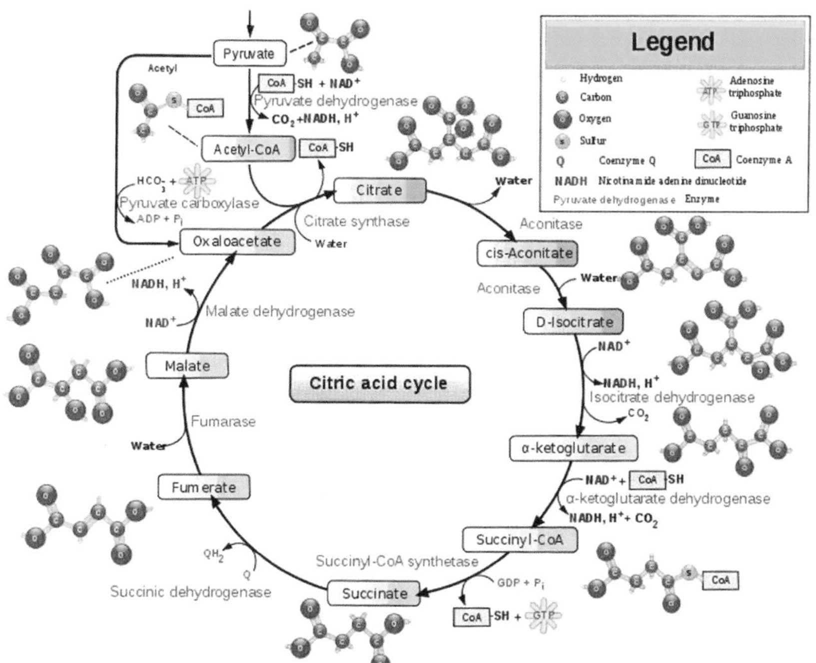

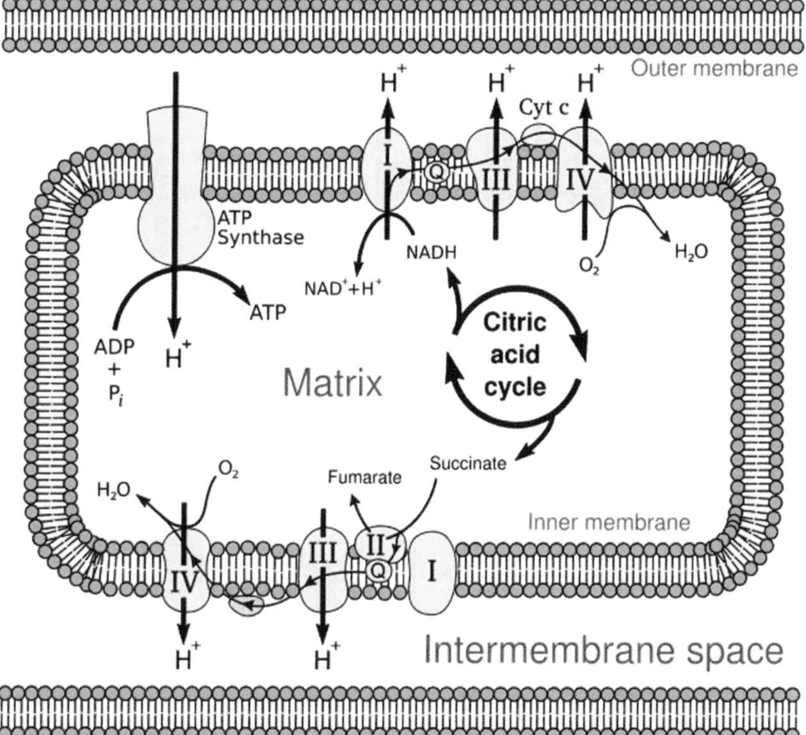

The Fate of Glucose

Glycolysis / Krebs cycle	Glycogen synthesis	Pentose-Phosphate Shunt
ATP CO_2 H_2O	Glycogen	Ribose CO_2 NADPH

(see text, page 187)

Vitamin	Biochemical action	Biological Role
B1 (thiamine)	Decarboxylation reactions - Release of CO2 in glycolysis, kreb's cycle and transketolase reactions	Glucose and Amino Acid metabolism
B2 (riboflavin)	Electron transport – Oxidation/Reduction	Glucose metabolism
B3 (Niacin)	Electron transport – Oxidation/Reduction	Glucose metabolism
B5 (Pantothenic Acid)	Component of CoA	Glucose and fatty acid metabolism, cholesterol synthesis
B6 (Pyridoxine)	Decarboxylation and Transamination	Amino acid metabolism
B12 (Cobalbumin)	1-Carbon metabolism	Nucleotide Synthesis, cysteine / methionine metabolism
Folic Acid	1-Carbon metabolism	Nucleotide Synthesis, cysteine / methionine metabolism
Biotin	Transcarboxylation reactions	Glucose, fatty acid, amino acid metabolism
C	Copper and Iron containing Hydroxylases	Fatty acid metabolism, Antioxidant
A	Active site of rhodopsin and iodopsin	Vision
D	Calcium and phosphorus metabolism	Bone and muscle strength, immune system modulation
E	Precise biochemical function unknown	Antioxidant
K	Protein carboxylation	Blood clotting factors, bone matrix synthesis

1.

Mineral	Biological Role
Calcium	Structure of bones, signal transduction, blood clotting
Chloride	Fluid and electrolyte balance
Chromium	Insulin sensitivity
Copper	Presence in the active site of enzymes
Iodine	Synthesis of thyroid hormone
Iron	Reversible oxygen binding in hemoglobin and myoglobin, oxidative phosphorylation enzymes
Magnesium	Presence in the active site of enzymes
Manganese	Presence in the active site of enzymes
Molybdenum	Presence in the active site of enzymes
Potassium	Nerve signal transduction
Selenium	Component of selenoproteins, free radical scavenger
Sodium	Fluid and electrolyte balance, nerve signal transduction
Zinc	Presence in the active site of enzymes, formation of zinc fingers

2.

Chapter 5.2

The Physiology of Nutrition

Jason M Hollander, MD, CNSP

Hunger and Satiety

An area of the brain known as the "hypothalamus" serves as the principle coordinator of eating behavior. The hypothalamus resides just above the pituitary gland, or "master gland," and essentially integrates information from the environment via sensory organs and the cerebral cortex, and from our internal physiology via our immune system and hormones. At one time, it was believed that meal onset was simply stimulated by the hypothalamus in response to the drop in blood sugar (glucose) between meals. However, more recent evidence suggests that meals are started primarily as a function of social and environmental influences. In other words, we eat when it is "lunch hour" and not so much because of complex biochemical messages related to blood glucose levels or our state of energy balance. Therefore, if not entirely controlled by when to start a meal, energy balance must be maintained by also knowing when to stop a meal. To this end, the hypothalamus creates the sensation of being satisfied or "full" ("satiety") so that energy intake is appropriate for the body's energy needs. This very complicated mechanism is still being unraveled by medical researchers and will ultimately result in the understanding of metabolic disorders and the development of effective medications for their treatment.

Peripheral Satiety Signals

The Gastrointestinal (GI) Tract

The GI tract generates a number of satiety signals in response to feeding. When nutrients enter the lumen of the GI tract, several proteins are released. These small molecules can circulate via the bloodstream and act directly on the hypothalamus. Additionally, these proteins trigger a series of nerve impulses by attaching to other proteins (called "receptors") on cells. These impulses carry vital information about energy intake to the hypothalamus. Some of the most important proteins are "cholecystokinin" (CCK), "glucagon-like peptide 1" (GLP-1), "peptide YY" (PYY), and "ghrelin."

CCK is made by cells in the small intestine and binds to nearby receptors delivering a message of fullness to the brain. Under some conditions, CCK can reduce meal size in various species of animals.

GLP-1 is another gut protein that is released in response to food intake. It has several important effects, including: 1) increased insulin production in response to increasing blood glucose levels, 2) delayed emptying of stomach contents, 3) decreased production of another protein called "glucagon" (a hormone from the pancreas that has opposite effects of insulin), and 4) increased message for fullness or satiety. A form of this protein hormone is known as "exenatide," which is an approved medication for diabetes. Exenatide also causes modest weight loss.

PYY is made by cells at the end of the small intestine in response to food. Scientific studies show that PYY reduces food intake in obese animals, but it is not known exactly how this happens. It is believed that PYY works on the hypothalamus.

Ghrelin is a gut hormone that can stimulate appetite. It is released from specialized cells in the stomach and acts on ghrelin receptors in the hypothalamus. Ghrelin levels increase prior to a meal and fall sharply following a meal. The control of ghrelin may be abnormal in some obese people. In other words, ghrelin may not decrease appropriately following a meal, so appetite would remain high and excess weight gain could occur. Recent research suggests that ghrelin responses may differ in response to intakes of carbohydrate, fat, and protein. Interestingly, blocking the ghrelin receptor does not seem to reduce appetite.

Fat Tissue

"Leptin" is another protein produced primarily in fat ("adipose") tissue. Leptin circulates in the bloodstream and enters the brain. Leptin plays an important role in the regulation of adipose tissue. It is also involved in regulating food intake and meal size. The genetic absence of leptin leads to severe obesity, which can be reduced by using leptin as a medicine. Unfortunately, leptin deficiency is a very rare disorder and does not explain the epidemic of obesity around the world.

Central Satiety Signals

A number of peptides produced and released in the central nervous system also convey important messages regarding energy balance to the hypothalamus for processing. Neuropeptide Y (NPY) is one of many peptides that increase appetite. This hormone is released when leptin levels are low, glucose levels are low, insulin levels are low, and under conditions of decreased food intake. When NPY is infused into the central nervous systems of rats, food intake is increased.

Pro-opiomelanocortin (POMC), on the other hand, decreases appetite. When rats are overfed, POMC levels increase and loss of appetite results. This pattern can be reversed by blocking receptors for POMC. In humans, as many as 5 percent of cases of severe obesity are associated with abnormalities in the POMC receptor.

Other neurotransmitters like norepinephrine, serotonin, and dopamine also participate in the regulation of feeding behavior. Serotonin, for instance, decreases food intake and body weight by decreasing appetite and increasing energy expenditure. Certain medications increase serotonin levels and have proven benefit in inducing weight loss in humans.

Integration of Multiple Signals

The messengers discussed above are just a handful of the countless inputs that control hunger and satiety. Central and peripheral signals are evaluated together, or integrated, in the hypothalamus, where an answer is produced in the form of "appetite." Since there are many signals, this system can rapidly adjust for changes in any one piece of the puzzle. This ultimately guarantees an adequate energy balance. The many backup systems that play a role, however, also explain why efforts to block appetite stimulation have such limited effect on body weight and composition.

The Physiologic Fate of Food

When food enters the mouth, digestion begins. Food is chewed, and saliva is produced in large quantities. Saliva moistens the food and contains digestive enzymes such as amylase, which begins to break down carbohydrates. The food is softened into a mass that can be swallowed. Then, the food travels down the esophagus into the stomach.

Once in the stomach, the food is thoroughly mixed with gastric acid and digestive enzymes. The acid provides the optimum environment for the enzyme pepsin to act. Pepsin works by breaking down proteins. Food is then passed through the stomach into the small intestine. The majority of digestion and absorption occurs here in the small intestine. The food mixture is now known as "chyme." Here, the chyme is mixed with bile, from the gallbladder, which allows for the absorption of fat and neutralizes the acid from the stomach. The chyme is also mixed with pancreatic and intestinal enzymes like maltase, lactase, sucrase, trypsin, and chymotrypsin. These enzymes break down proteins and carbohydrates into their building block parts to make absorption of these nutrients easier.

Nutrients can then pass through the intestinal wall along finger-like projections called "villi." The blood that absorbs the nutrients is carried directly to the liver through the "portal vein." The liver filters the blood, removing toxins and processing nutrients. The remaining material in the small intestine moves along by peristalsis (rhythmic contractions of the intestinal walls). Ultimately, the food passes from the small intestine to the large intestine. The large intestine absorbs water and stores the fecal waste until it can be eliminated as a bowel movement.

Hormonal Control of Nutrient Metabolism

Once the nutrients reach the liver, hormonal signals determine the economy of nutrition, that is, which calories are to be burned immediately and which are to be saved for future use. In the fed state, specialized cells in the pancreas known as "beta-cells" sense glucose levels rising and release insulin, a hormone with multiple actions throughout the body.

- Insulin acts on the liver cells and muscle cells to stimulate glucose uptake.
- Once energy requirements are met, insulin signals the storage of excess carbohydrate as "glycogen."
- Insulin stimulates fat (adipose) tissue to take up free fatty acids in the bloodstream and store them in the form of triglycerides.
- Insulin decreases the breakdown of protein ("proteolysis") and the breakdown of fat ("lipolysis").
- Insulin decreases the process of "gluconeogenesis"—the mechanism by which non-glucose molecules are converted into glucose during fasting (so that the body always has

a constant supply of glucose, even with starvation).

Between meals, insulin levels begin to drop. Naturally, in the fasting state, energy must be released from bodily stores to ensure a steady current of energy to the brain, muscles, and other vital organs. As insulin's cell-building, or anabolic, effects are withdrawn, glycogen is broken down into glucose, in a process known as glycogenolysis. Free fatty acids are released from adipose tissue by lipolysis, and amino acids are released by proteolysis.

Simultaneously, glucagon levels begin to rise. Glucagon is released during fasting by the "alpha-cells" of the pancreas. Its effects are directly opposite of the effects of insulin. Glucagon signals the liver to break down glycogen into glucose and to initiate gluconeogenesis, if necessary, to maintain glucose balance in the body. Glucagon also stimulates the release of free fatty acids, which can be converted into ketones and burned as fuel. It is important to note that re-directing the flow of food energy from muscle (protein) and adipose tissue (fat) into glucose during starvation comes with a price: decreased muscle mass and decreased fat mass. This is why we become "skinny" when we fast or starve. In short, the body is able to guarantee a steady energy supply to support vital functions and activity, regardless of daily energy intake, and this is managed by hormones.

Conclusions

A complex set of signals bombards the hypothalamus, which integrates the information and determines if energy intake is sufficient. When energy intake is sufficient, satiety ensues. Under the regulation of glucagon and insulin, the calories that are consumed are processed and either used now or later depending on feeding patterns and energy expenditure. These complex systems guarantee that energy will be available at all times to support vital functions and daily activities.

Selected Readings

Atkinson TF. Central and peripheral neuroendocrine peptides and signaling in appetite regulation: considerations for obesity pharmacotherapy. Obes Rev. 2008; 9:108–120.

Chaudhri OB, Wynne K, Bloom SR. Can gut hormones control appetite and prevent obesity? Diabetes Care. 2008; 31. (Supp 2):S284–89.

Crowley VE. Overview of human obesity and central mechanisms regulating energy homeostasis. Ann Clin Biochem. 2008; 45:245–55.

Shils ME, Shike M, Ross AC, et al. (eds). *Modern Nutrition in Health and Disease,* 10th Edition. Lippincott Williams & Wilkins, New York, 2006.

Valassi E, Scacchi M, Cavagnini F. Neuroendocrine control of food intake. Nutr Metab Cardiovasc Dis. 2008; 18:158–68.

Chapter 5.3

Nutrient-gene Interactions

Yi-Hao Yu, MD, PhD, FACE, CNSP

The classical nutrient-gene interactions are exemplified by the discoveries of some single-gene diseases. People who have these diseases can be helped by the elimination, restriction, or supplementation of specific nutritional components in the diet. For example, mutations in the gene for "branched-chain alpha-ketoacid dehydrogenase" (BCKD) are the underlying problem for a genetic disease called "maple syrup urine disease" (MSUD). Individuals who have this rare genetic disease must be put on a special diet with minimal amounts of the branched-chain amino acids leucine, isoleucine, and valine in order to prevent neurological damage and live a normal life. As another example, mutations in the gene for the "low density lipoprotein receptor" (LDLR) or in the gene for "apolipoprotein B" cause "familial hypercholesterolemia" (FH). In addition to drug and other special therapies, individuals who are afflicted with this hereditary disease must be put on a diet that is largely depleted of saturated fats, *trans* fats, and cholesterol.

Common diseases are generally multifactorial in nature and involve multiple layers of interactions between genetic and environmental factors. These diseases include obesity, type 2 diabetes, the metabolic syndrome, cardiovascular disease, and cancer.

While "nutrigenetics" is the study of nutrient-gene interactions at the gene level, "nutrigenomics" is the study of nutrient-gene interactions at the genome (the whole set of human genes) level. Individuals have different forms or variants of the same genes; this is called "genetic polymorphism." Therefore, the outcomes of nutrient-gene interactions are different in different individuals. Moreover, nutritional care must be individualized in order to effectively prevent disease and promote health.

The concept of "personalized nutrition" or "individualized nutrition" is analogous to that of "personalized medicine" or "individualized medicine" in which an individual's genetic makeup is considered a critical determinant that predicts responses to nutrition or drug therapy, respectively. Both concepts are born of, and rapidly facilitated in their development by, the Human Genome Project and the systemic search and identification of gene polymorphisms, including numerous "single nucleotide polymorphisms" (SNPs). Future nutrigenetic and nutrigenomic research holds promise for individualized nutrition that will deliver more effective diagnostic, preventive, and treatment options for common chronic diseases.

In the following sections, instead of providing an exhaustive collection of research data on nutrient-gene interactions, we will use a few examples related to two common diseases, lipid disorders and cancer, to illustrate how nutrient-gene interactions work and how the research in this field may ultimately lead to individualized nutrition. Interested readers may also refer to the references list at the end of the chapter for more advanced reading and study of the relevant research data.

Nutrient-gene Interactions in Lipid Disorders and Atherosclerosis

"Atherosclerosis" is a condition in which arterial blood vessels are "hardened" by lipid deposition ("plaques") with inflammation inside the vessel wall. The passageway of the affected blood vessels is narrowed by the plaques, causing insufficient blood supply to the area fed by the affected vessels. Complete blockage of a vessel can occur when the plaques are ruptured, which elicits a host of biochemical reactions that lead to the clotting. Atherosclerosis is considered a key element of cardiovascular disease, heart attack, stroke, and other peripheral artery occlusive diseases.

Major risk factors for atherosclerosis include high blood levels of LDL-cholesterol ("bad" cholesterol), high blood levels of triglyceride, and low blood levels of HDL-cholesterol ("good" cholesterol). "Apolipoproteins" are the protein components of lipoprotein particles that carry cholesterol, triglyceride, and other lipids in the circulation, and various apolipoproteins are encoded by corresponding genes such as APOA1, APOC3, APOA4, and others.

The levels of blood lipids are influenced by both genetic and dietary factors. The combination of an individual's genetic makeup and dietary habits predicts the outcome. People who carry the gene variant (or "allele" in genetic terms) for APOA1*A allele (as opposed to the APOA1*G allele) will usually have elevated blood LDL-cholesterol levels if they consume a fat-rich diet. An allele is one member of a pair of DNA sequences that make up a gene. Similarly, people who carry the APOA4*2 allele (as opposed to the APOA4*1 allele) will be at higher risk for lipid-related cardiovascular diseases if they smoke cigarettes and eat fat-rich foods. Those who carry the APOC3*S2 allele (as opposed to the APOC3*S1 allele) may have higher blood levels of cholesterol and triglyceride, but they may lower their LDL-cholesterol levels by increasing the amount of monounsaturated fat in their diet.

The "lipoprotein lipase" (LPL) gene offers another good example in this category. This gene has two variants that differ in the regulatory region of the gene, "H-" and "H+." People who carry the H- variant may significantly improve their blood triglyceride levels by consuming foods high in polyunsaturated fats (e.g., vegetable oil) and low in saturated fats (e.g., animal fat). However, this type of dietary intervention has very limited effect on people who carry the H+ allele.

Finally, the "apolipoprotein E" (APOE) gene, which encodes a common protein found in several lipoprotein particles, has three common variants—"e2," "e3," and "e4"—that are defined by different combinations of two SNPs within the gene. People who have the e2 or e4 variants are associated with a higher risk for developing lipid disorders and cardiovascular disease, especially when combined with diets rich in fat. Interestingly, the e4 variant also put the carriers at a higher risk for developing Alzheimer's disease later in life, although the significance of this nutrient-gene interaction here is currently unclear.

Nutrient-gene Interactions in Cancer Development

The importance of diet and environmental factors in the prevention and development of cancer is being increasingly recognized. Lack of dietary fiber, deficiency in folic acid, and an excess of saturated fat all have been associated with certain types of cancer. Obviously, not all people develop cancer even when they eat the same "bad" food and live in the same environment.

In other words, because of the differences in genetic makeup, gene-environment interactions, and gene-nutrient interactions, some people may, more than others, be susceptible to developing certain types of cancer by eating certain types of food. On the other hand, some types of food may be protective against certain types of cancer to some people and have no effect in others.

How does diet modify the risk of cancer, and how is this related to genetic polymorphism? Even though nutrient-gene interactions are, in general, less well-characterized in cancer biology than are those in lipid and cardiovascular biology, such interactions are believed to be universally present. For example, certain types of breast and prostate cancers are promoted by sex hormones. Many foods contain various types of steroids or precursors of sex hormones. Genetic polymorphisms exist in genes involved in the synthesis and metabolism of steroids and sex hormones, such as the 5α-reductase type 2, 3β-hydroxysteroid dehydrogenase, and catechol-O-methyltransferase genes. Thus, depending on an individual's genetic makeup, steroidal substrates in food may be converted to effective carcinogens in some people but not in others. Additionally, the genes for sex hormone receptors are polymorphic, which implies that the sensitivity of an individual to hormonal stimulation of tumor growth varies greatly.

An example of relatively well-characterized nutrient-gene interactions in cancer biology is the interactions of the nutritional components folate and alcohol with the gene encoding the enzyme "5,10-methylenetetrahydrofolate reductase" (MTHFR). Folate-deficient diet and alcohol consumption have been linked to colorectal cancers in some patients. How do nutrients interact with the MTHFR gene with respect to the risk for colorectal cancers? This has to do with a chemical process termed "DNA methylation." Since DNA methylation does not alter the genetic codes per se, but silences the expression of the DNA codes, it is regarded as an "epigenetic" phenomenon (not directly affecting the gene sequence). Globally *impaired* DNA methylation or gene-silencing programs can cause developmental abnormalities or lead to cancer growth in rapidly growing tissues such as in the colon or rectum. Several important factors are involved in the DNA methylation process. "S-adenosyl-l-methionine" is the methyl donor used for DNA methylation. MTHFR is required for the synthesis of this methyl donor, and folate is another regulator in these multi-step biochemical reactions. If dietary folate is deficient, then the synthesis and availability of the methyl donor will be reduced, and as a result, DNA methylation will be *impaired.*

Global DNA hypomethylation is not the only factor frequently associated with tumor cell development; when the MTHFR-mediated biochemical reaction is slowed, the intermediate metabolites "methyltetrahydrofolate" and "methylenetetrahydrofolate," two molecules regarded as carcinogenic in the development of colorectal cancers, will accumulate. Thus, people who carry the particular MTHFR gene variant (C677T) have reduced MTHFR enzyme activities and will be at higher risk for colorectal cancer, especially if they eat a folate-poor diet. The combination of this particular MTHFR gene variant and a folate-poor diet puts them at a high risk for colorectal cancer. These patients exhibit impaired DNA methylation and high levels of the intermediate metabolites, which are reflected by elevated blood levels of the amino acid "homocysteine," a clinical biomarker measurable in the blood to indicate impaired DNA methylation. On the other hand, people who carry two copies of the "C" variant of the MTHFR gene are less affected by the dietary folate levels because of the highly active enzyme that they have inherited.

Alcohol comes into play by indirectly affecting the absorption and metabolism of folate as well as by interfering with the synthesis of the methyl donor. Alcohol blocks the release of folate from the liver, thus reducing the effective bioavailability of dietary folate. Alcohol can also deplete the body's folate stores by interfering with the absorption and cellular retention of folate through some of the alcohol metabolites. In addition, alcohol inhibits methyl donor synthesis through the alcohol metabolite "acetaldehyde." Therefore, a low-folate diet plus alcohol is regarded as a carcinogenic methyl-deficient diet, particularly for people with the C677T MTHFR gene variant.

Take-home Messages

So, what can the above examples of nutrient-gene interactions tell us? Should we be overly concerned about what gene variants we carry? Should we feel doomed if we happen to carry some "undesirable" gene variants, but be elated and think we can forget about good nutritional and healthy lifestyle practices if we happen to inherit some "desirable" gene variants? Of course, the answer is "no."

First of all, the many different gene variants being discussed are common gene variants, not rare gene mutations. The gene variants should not be considered as disease-causing or non-disease-causing genes. Instead, they should be regarded as genetic elements that may put someone at higher risks for developing certain diseases. This distinction is important because not all people who have a disease-susceptible gene variant develop the disease, and not all people who develop the disease have the specific disease-susceptible gene variant.

Secondly, the above examples should reinforce the concept of healthy eating for everyone. Until we have more complete knowledge about the vast complexities of all human nutrient-gene interactions, there can be no certainty about a person's risk or individualized optimal diet. For example, people who have the APOA1*G gene variant are less affected by dietary fats, but it does not mean they should not watch out for cardiovascular disease associated with fat-rich diets. This is because the risk factors for cardiovascular disease or other diseases are not determined solely by one or several gene variants, but by many more factors, many of which are yet to be learned. So, common sense for healthy eating and balanced diets still prevails over the incomplete knowledge of whether or not one carries one or more low-risk gene variants. Besides, to make the matter more complex, a certain gene variant may confer a high risk for one disease but a low risk for another disease. For example, the APOE e4 gene variant confers a higher risk for developing breast cancer in women who have high blood triglyceride levels, but it may protect them against colon cancer. So, it is wise not to deviate from a healthy eating practice.

These being said, the examples of nutrient-gene interactions do illustrate the concept that if we knew all about nutrient-gene interactions regarding a particular set of gene variants in relation to certain diets and certain diseases, then we ought to be able to make a very intelligent dietary recommendation based on any individual's genetic makeup. This is exactly the promise of the nutrigenetics and nutrigenomics research—the futuristic "designer diets" that are aimed at preemptively offsetting the diseases to which certain individuals may be genetically susceptible. This is the exciting part of nutritional research.

Suggested readings

Adlercreutz H. Phyto-oestrogens and cancer. Lancet Oncol, 2002; 3:364-373.

Chen J, Ma J, Stampfer MJ, Palomeque C, Selhub J, and Hunter DJ. Linkage disequilibrium between the 677C>T and 1298A>C polymorphisms in human methylenetetrahydrofolate reductase gene and their contributions to risk of colorectal cancer. Pharmacogenetics, 2002; 12:339-342.

DeBusk RM, Fogarty CP, Ordovas JM, and Kornman KS. Nutritional genomics in practice: where do we begin? J Am Diet Assoc, 2005; 105:589-598.

Dunning AM, Healey CS, Pharoah, PD, Teare MD, Ponder BA, and Easton DF. A systematic review of genetic polymorphisms and breast cancer risk. Cancer Epidemiol Biomarkers Prev 8, 1999; 843-854.

Friso S, Choi SW , Girelli D, Mason JB, Dolnikowski GG, Bagley PJ, Olivieri O, Jacques PF, Rosenberg IH, Corrocher R, et al. A common mutation in the 5,10-methylenetetrahydrofolate reductase gene affects genomic DNA methylation through an interaction with folate status. Proc Natl Acad Sci U S A, 2002; 99:5606-5611.

Go VL, Wong DA, Wang Y, Butrum RR, Norman HA, and Wilkerson L. Diet and cancer prevention: evidence-based medicine to genomic medicine. J Nutr, 2004; 134:3513S-3516S.

Groenendijk M, Cantor RM, de Bruin TW , and Dallinga-Thie GM. The apoAI-CIII-AIV gene cluster. Atherosclerosis, 2001; 157:1-11.

Hanson NQ, Aras O, Yang F, and Tsai MY. C677T and A1298C polymorphisms of the methylenetetrahydrofolate reductase gene: incidence and effect of combined genotypes on plasma fasting and post-methionine load homocysteine in vascular disease. Clin Chem, 2001; 47:661-666.

Kervinen K, Sodervik H, Makela J, Lehtola J, Niemi M, Kairaluoma MI, and Kesaniemi YA. Is the development of adenoma and carcinoma in proximal colon related to apolipoprotein E phenotype? Gastroenterology,1996; 110:1785-1790.

Loktionov A. Common gene polymorphisms and nutrition: emerging links with pathogenesis of multifactorial chronic diseases (review). J Nutr Biochem, 2003; 14:426-451.

Molloy AM, and Scott JM. Folates and prevention of disease. Public Health Nutr, 2001; 4:601-609.

Moysich KB, Freudenheim JL, Baker JA, Ambrosone CB, Bowman ED, Schisterman, EF, Vena, JE, and Shields PG. Apolipoprotein E genetic polymorphism, serum lipoproteins, and breast cancer risk. Mol Carcinog, 2007; 27:2-9.

Nwosu V, Carpten J, Trent JM, and Sheridan R. Heterogeneity of genetic alterations in prostate cancer: evidence of the complex nature of the disease. Hum Mol Genet, 2001; 10:2313-2318.

Ordovas JM, and Schaefer EJ. Genetic determinants of plasma lipid response to dietary intervention: the role of the APOA1/C3/A4 gene cluster and the APOE gene. Br J Nutr, 2000; 83:S127-136.

Ordovas JM, Corella D, Cupples LA, Demissie S, Kelleher A, Coltell O, Wilson PW , Schaefer EJ, and Tucker K. Polyunsaturated fatty acids modulate the effects of the APOA1 G-A polymorphism on HDL-cholesterol concentrations in a sex-specific manner: The Framingham Study. Am J Clin Nutr, 2002; 75:38-46.

Shannon B, Gnanasampanthan S, Beilby J, and Iacopetta B. A polymorphism in the methylenetetrahydrofolate reductase gene predisposes to colorectal cancers with microsatellite instability. Gut, 2002; 50:520-524.

Song C, Xing D, Tan W , Wei Q, and Lin D. Methylenetetrahydrofolate reductase polymorphisms increase risk of esophageal squamous cell carcinoma in a Chinese population. Cancer Res, 2001; 61:3272-3275.

Stover PJ Influence of human genetic variation on nutritional requirements. Am J Clin Nutr, 2006; 83:436S-442S.

Subbiah MT. Nutrigenetics and nutraceuticals: the next wave riding on personalized medicine. Transl Res, 2007; 149:55-61.

Watson MA, Gay L, Stebbings WS, Speakman CT, Bingham SA, and Loktionov A. Apolipoprotein E gene polymorphism and colorectal cancer: Gender-specific modulation of risk and prognosis. Clin Sci (Lond), 2003; 104:537-545.

Chapter 5.4

Future Developments in Nutritional Medicine

Jeffrey I. Mechanick, MD, FACP, FACE, FACN
Elise M. Brett, MD, FACE, CNSP

Advances in nutritional medicine have traditionally lagged behind advances in other medical fields. For the most part, current research into various diseases does not uniformly incorporate nutritional causes and treatments. On the other hand, within the realm of preventive medicine, nutritional medicine has kept pace with other disciplines. Furthermore, as disease mechanisms are clarified and their primary treatments become more effective, overall longevity, quality of life, and healthy aging surface as high priorities for the public. How might future nutritional interventions ultimately impact the prevention and treatment of disease? Two examples are given below.

Future Nutritional Intervention #1: Genetically-engineered Foods

Genetic engineering is capable of producing "genetically modified foods" from genetically modified organisms. This is accomplished by taking one organism's DNA, changing it in the laboratory so that a new or improved function will result, and then inserting it into the target organism's genome so that the resulting plant or animal will provide a superior food. Other techniques that can produce beneficial results involve increasing or decreasing copies of certain genes, silencing or removing certain genes, or modifying the position of certain genes within the genome.

Potential benefits include prolonged shelf life; better taste and flavor; resistance to pests, disease, and other infections; tolerance to herbicides or other chemical exposures; tolerance to adverse climatic conditions; quicker maturation and greater food yield; and incorporation of bioactive substances that confer a nutritional or medicinal advantage. Some foods that are genetically engineered include corn, soybean, rapeseed, tomato, potato, rice, cantaloupe, sugar beet, radicchio, flax, papaya, squash, and alfalfa. In America, genetically engineered foods are not labeled.

Critics of genetically engineered foods argue that potential adverse health consequences cannot be predicted, environmental safety is compromised, and that this methodology is just not necessary to solve the world's nutrition problems. If the contentious issues surrounding genetically engineered foods can be resolved, the future may witness the incorporation of various pharmaceuticals, such as vaccines, into various foods. Applied safely and systematically to populations at risk, this technology could prevent disease, improve health, and extend life.

Future Nutritional Intervention #2: Nutrigenomics

Another bright spot on the horizon for nutrition is the field of "nutrigenomics." This fairly new discipline deals with the interface between the human genome and nutritional factors. One can envision a future wherein personalized medicine is the standard. In other words, every human being's genomic makeup will be characterized at or even before birth and then stored using advanced bioinformatics. Research will have identified a host of nutrient-gene interactions that identify disease risk; lead to disease prevention, treatment, and cure; and improve physical and cognitive performance. Clinical and mathematical algorithms will then design personalized diets and meal plans for individuals, perhaps even from shortly after conception. In chapter 5.3, "Nutrient-Gene Interactions," several examples of potential nutrigenomic interventions were given; for example, a high polyunsaturated fat diet in people with the H- variant of the lipoprotein lipase gene to improve blood triglyceride levels, and folate supplementation in people with the C677T variant of the 5,10-methylenetetrahydrofolate reductase gene to reduce the risk for colorectal cancer.

To Review...

These are exciting times in medicine, and the responsibility for proper nutrition lies squarely with both the doctor and the patient. Each of us must endeavor to eat right and increase physical activity to improve our lives. The messages of each of the chapters in this book converge on a simple set of priorities. It is not important to be perfect or to adhere exactly to the recommendations, but it is important to reflect on the many priorities in life and the role of a healthy lifestyle.

CHAPTER 5.5

A Call for Action

Elise M. Brett, MD, FACE, CNSP
Jeffrey I. Mechanick, MD, FACP, FACE, FACN

This book describes what healthy eating is all about. Despite the explosion of fad diets and multiple, diverse published statements on what a healthy diet should be, the final common denominator among scientifically based nutritional recommendations is a plant-based diet with high fiber, phytonutrients, mono- and polyunsaturated fats, and high biological quality protein. There is plenty of room for variation based on genetics, existing medical conditions, ethnic and cultural diversity, and even personal preferences. If more people would follow a healthy eating plan, it is likely that the prevalence of certain diseases in this country would decrease and the monetary cost to our society would be reduced. Yet people are slow in adopting a healthy eating program. We believe that the government, those in the food business, and those in leadership positions in certain other businesses can intervene at various levels to help implement the healthy diet prescription described in this book.

For many people, eating healthier means a major lifestyle change. However, changing old habits is difficult. This usually means making better food choices. It may mean more frequent shopping to ensure having fresh produce, fish, and meats at home. It may also mean advanced planning, like preparing lunch at home and bringing it to work to avoid eating the most readily available fast food.

It would be best to develop good eating habits early in life and not to have to make these changes later on. Children as young as kindergarten age can learn about making good food choices. Nutrition education should begin in our schools in kindergarten and continue through grade school to reinforce and expand upon basic principles. School cafeterias should provide healthy, well-balanced meals that encourage the choosing of foods from each of the different food groups. The government may need to provide increased funding so that school cafeterias can cook and serve unprocessed foods, preferably incorporating local produce. Candy, sodas, potato chips, and other "junk foods" with little nutritional value should be kept out of schools. Parents would be wise to avoid the concept of "kid food" and encourage children to eat what they are eating. Many restaurants have children's menus with the same high-fat items such as fried chicken nuggets, pizza, hamburgers, and macaroni and cheese. Alternatively, restaurants could offer smaller portions or simpler versions of main menu items for children at a lower cost.

Private businesses, as well as hospitals and other public institutions, could choose to keep vending machines containing items with low nutritional value out of the buildings to avoid the temptation to buy these items as they are passed in the hall. Alternatively, they could insist that the machines carry only healthier options such as nuts, dried fruit, or low-fat pretzels. Some vending machines now sell refrigerated fresh items, like apples, bananas, and low-fat yogurts. These types of machines could be more widely used.

Overweight and obesity occur from caloric intake in excess of the body's requirements. Many people who are trying to lose weight or maintain weight loss are familiar with calorie counting. Calorie counting has become easier in recent years due to the requirements for Nutrition Facts labeling on packaged foods and easy access to this information on the Internet. Those who have tried counting calories know that the greatest challenge in calorie counting comes when eating out. Several counties in New York and California recently enacted laws requiring certain chain restaurants to post calorie information on their menus. Fewer people may choose to have that afternoon snack knowing that the calorie amount equals or exceeds one-quarter of their recommended daily caloric intake. People can use calorie information to make better choices among menu items. Furthermore, restaurants, knowing they need to post such information, may be encouraged to substitute certain ingredients for lower calorie options or to reduce portion sizes. More widespread implementation of such laws would facilitate healthy eating for the general public.

Restaurant management in general should reconsider portion sizes. Only in America does one frequently find such enormous portions (often enough for two or three people) or "all you can eat" buffets. Restaurants can fill the dinner plates by increasing portions of vegetables rather than having the steak or roast beef hanging off the side of the plate to show how much food is provided. Most people will eat what is put in front of them, rather than leaving food on the plate, even if they would have been satisfied with a smaller portion. The idea of "getting one's money's worth" by eating more per meal when eating out needs to change. There must be greater focus on quality rather than quantity. Restaurant management can focus their marketing and advertisements on a "healthier" meal rather than a "large" meal.

As discussed previously, *trans* fats are the unhealthiest types of fat and should be severely limited in or even excluded from the diet. The government has recently required the labeling of amounts of *trans* fat on packaged foods. New York City has taken this one step further and actually banned the sale of prepared foods containing more than 0.5 grams of *trans* fat per serving. Other local governments could follow suit. This would not harm sales for those in the food business, but would simply force changes to healthier ingredients.

Other measures such as an "obesity tax" on non-diet sodas and fruit drinks containing less than 70 percent fruit juice are now being considered and may discourage the consumption of these highly caloric, low nutritional quality beverages. It is not the type of sugar in these drinks (often high fructose corn syrup), but rather the excessive consumption of calories that results from inclusion of these products in the diet that has contributed to the epidemic of obesity in this country.

Most people enjoy fresh fruits and vegetables as part of their diets. The experience can be even more enjoyable when consuming local produce, which is often fresher and tastier, always seasonal, and may be available at lower cost. Supporting local farmers through programs that facilitate sales to local supermarkets is another set of measures that can promote healthy eating. Local governments can also encourage the organization of weekly "farmer's markets" in nearby cities to increase consumption of local produce at a lower cost due to minimal overhead and low transportation costs. The federal government could remove barriers to farmers who wish to plant new fruit and vegetable crops. This would also encourage the expansion of community-supported agriculture programs in which produce is sold in advance of the growing season and delivered on a weekly basis as crops become available. City governments can provide more permits for street vendors selling fresh fruits and vegetables as opposed to hot dogs and ice cream.

The cumulative effect of the above, and of course many other, initiatives can truly accelerate healthy eating and consequently greater overall health of the population. The American Association of Clinical Endocrinologists, American College of Endocrinology, along with other medical societies, have for a long time supported programs to educate and promote healthy eating, increased physical activity, and comprehensive health care to improve our lifestyles. What is needed now is a more aggressive commitment and approach from our leaders in government to support these measures. It is the hope of all the authors involved in this book that healthy eating by everyone becomes a reality.

Appendix I

Dietary Reference Intakes

Jeffrey I. Mechanick, MD, FACP, FACE, FACN

Prior to the 1990s, the way in which various nutrients were evaluated for healthy people was based on the Recommended Dietary Allowances (RDA). Now, these nutrients are evaluated based on a more specific set of guidelines termed the Dietary Reference Intakes (DRI). Instead of just the RDA classification of nutrients, there are now three other ways based on the amount and type of scientific information available. Various nutrients and the DRI values (based on all four ways, where applicable) are given in the following table.

Dietary Reference Intakes

Nutrient per day	RDA[1]	AI[2]	UL[3]	AMDR (%)[4]
Water (L)		2.1 – 3.3		
Sodium (g)		1.2 – 1.5	2.2 – 2.3	
Potassium (g)		4.5 – 4.7		
Protein (g)	34 – 56			10 – 35
Carbohydrate (g)	130			45 – 65
Fat (g)				25 - 35
Fiber (g)		21 – 38		
n-6 PUFA (g)		10 – 17		5 – 10
n-3 PUFA (g)		1.0 – 1.6		0.6 – 1.2
biotin (µg)		20 – 30		
choline (mg)		375 – 550	2000 – 3000	
folate (µg)	300 – 400		600 – 1000	
niacin (mg)	12 – 14		20 – 35	
pantothenic acid (mg)		4 – 5		
riboflavin (mg)	0.9 – 1.3			
thiamine (mg)	0.9 – 1.1			
vitamin A (µg)	600 – 900		1700 – 3000	
vitamin B6 (mg)	1.0 – 1.7		60 – 100	
vitamin B12 (µg)	1.8 – 2.4			
vitamin C (mg)	45 – 90		1200 – 2000	
vitamin D (µg)	5 – 15		50	
vitamin E (µg)	11 – 15		600 – 1000	
vitamin K (µg)		60 – 120		
boron (mg)			20-Nov	
calcium (mg)		1000 - 1300		
copper (µg)	700 – 900		5000 – 10000	
iron (µg)	120 – 150		600 – 1100	
magnesium (mg)	240 – 420		350	
molybdenum (µg)	34 – 45		1100 – 2000	
phosphorus (mg)	700 – 1250		3000 – 4000	
selenium (mg)	40 – 55		280 – 400	
vanadium (mg)			1.8	
zinc (mg)	8 – 11		23 – 40	

1 Recommended Daily Allowance (RDA) = average nutrient intake that meets the needs of 97–98 percent of healthy people

2 Adequate Intake (AI) = recommended nutrient intake when the RDA is not available

3 Tolerable Upper Intake Level (TUL) = highest safe level of daily nutrient intake

4 Acceptable Macronutrient Distribution Range (AMDR) = intake (as a percentage) associated with reduced risk for a chronic disease

Abbreviations: L – liters, g – grams, PUFA – polyunsaturated fatty acid

Appendix II

Nutrient Content of Common Foods

Jeffrey I. Mechanick, MD, FACP, FACE, FACN

As you review these tables, take note of the contents of the "healthy foods," among which are fresh or fiber-containing frozen fruits and vegetables, seafood, whole grains, various monounsaturated plant oils, and low- or no-fat dairy products. The nutrient amounts in the second column for each table should be compared with the Dietary Reference Intake amounts provided in chapter 6.1. In addition, you should recognize the usual serving sizes listed. For instance, healthy meat portions are generally 3 ounces and grains ½ cup. Portion control is a very important part of a healthy meal plan and overall diet, especially when trying to achieve and maintain a healthy weight. It is also useful to see the effects of cooking (raw, baked, or boiled), food preparation (peel on or off), and varying fat content (dairy products and beef) on the various nutrient amounts. Several references are given at the end of this chapter, but if nutritional detail is desired for any particular food, the "Nutrition Data" Web site will be very useful (http://www.nutritiondata.com/). Items that are "POWER OF PREVENTION Healthy Foods" or related foods that are discussed in chapter 2.6 are in **bold**. In general, these will include low-fat dairy products, fish, eggs, and virtually all plant products (except for fruit juices). Remember, there are no absolutely "good" or "bad" foods, but rather "healthy" foods that are recommended to make up the bulk of your daily eating.

There are several abbreviations that are used in this chapter:

- "g" = grams
- "mg" = milligrams (1000 mg = 1 g)
- "mcg" = micrograms (1000 mcg = 1 mg)
- "oz" = ounce
- "tsp" = teaspoon
- "tbsp" = tablespoon

Protein Rich Foods	**Protein (g)**
Cottage cheese, low-fat, 1 cup	**28.1**
Hamburger, extra lean, 3 oz	24.3
Chicken roasted, 3 oz	21.3
Tuna, water packed, 3 oz	**20.1**
Beefsteak, broiled, 3 oz	19.3
Cheese pizza, 2 slices	15.4
Yogurt, low fat, 8 oz	**11.9**
Tofu, ½ cup	**10.1**
Lentils, cooked, ½ cup	**9**
Milk, skim, 8 oz	**8.4**
Split peas, cooked, ½ cup	**8.1**
Milk, whole, 8 oz	8
Corn, cooked, ½ cup	8.0
Lentil soup, 1 cup	**7.8**
Kidney beans, cooked, ½ cup	**7.6**
Cheddar cheese, 1 oz	7.1
Potato, baked with skin, large	7.0
Macaroni, cooked, 1 cup	6.8
Soymilk, 1 cup	**6.7**
Egg, large	**6.3**
Bread, whole-wheat, 2 slices	5.4
Bread, white, 2 slices	4.9
Rice, cooked, 1 cup	4.3
Broccoli, cooked, 1 cup	**2.6**

Fat-Containing Foods	Saturated Fat Content (g)
Dairy	
Regular cheddar cheese, 1 oz	6.0
Low-fat cheddar cheese, 1 oz	1.2
Whole milk (3.25%), 1 cup	4.6
Low-fat (1%) milk, 1 cup	1.5
Regular ice cream, ½ cup	4.9
Frozen yogurt, low-fat, ½ cup	2.0
Butter, 1 tsp	2.4
Soft Margarine with no *trans* fats, 1 tsp	0.7
Meat	
Regular ground beef (25% fat), 3 oz cooked	6.1
Extra Lean ground Beef (5%), 3 oz cooked	2.6
Fried chicken leg with Skin, 3 oz cooked	
Roasted chicken breast without skin, 3 oz cooked	
Breads	
Croissant, 1 medium	6.6
Bagel, oat bran, 1 medium 4"	0.2

Type of Fat	Main Food Sources
Monounsaturated	olives
	oils (canola, olive, peanut)
	nuts (cashew, almond, peanut, other nuts)
	avocado
Polyunsaturated	fish
	oils (corn, cottonseed, safflower, soybean)
Saturated	dairy (whole milk, butter, cheese, ice cream)
	red meat
	chocolate
	coconut, coconut milk and coconut oil
Trans	most margarines
	vegetable shortening
	partially hydrogenated vegetable oil
	deep-fried chips
	many snack foods and fast foods
	most commercial baked goods

Fiber Rich Foods		Dietary Fiber (g)
Navy beans, cooked, ½ cup		9.5
Bran cereal (100%), ready-to-eat, ½ cup		8.8
Kidney beans, canned, ½ cup		8.2
Split peas, cooked, ½ cup		8.1
Lentils, cooked, ½ cup		7.8
Black beans, cooked, ½ cup		7.5
Pinto beans, cooked ½ cup		7.7
Lima beans, cooked, ½ cup		6.6
Artichoke, globe, cooked		6.5
White beans, canned, ½ cup		6.3
Chickpeas, cooked, ½ cup		6.2
Great northern beans, cooked, ½ cup		6.2
Cowpeas, cooked, ½ cup		5.6
Soybeans, mature, cooked, ½ cup		5.2
Rye wafer crackers, plain, 2		5
Sweet potato, baked with peel, medium		4.8
Asian pear, raw, small		4.4
Green peas, cooked, ½ cup		4.4
English muffin, whole-wheat		4.4
Pear, raw, small		4.3
Bulgur, cooked, ½ cup		4.1
Mixed vegetables, cooked, ½ cup		4
Raspberries, raw, ½ cup		4
Sweet potato, boiled, no peel, medium		3.8
Blackberries, raw, ½ cup		3.8
Potato, baked, with skin, medium		3.8
Soybeans, green, cooked, ½ cup		3.8
Stewed prunes, ½ cup		3.8
Figs, dried, ¼ cup		3.7
Dates, ¼ cup		3.6
Oat bran, raw, ¼ cup		3.6
Pumpkin, canned, ½ cup		3.6
Spinach, cooked from frozen, ½ cup		3.5
Shredded wheat cereal, ready-to-eat, about 1 oz		2.8 to 3.4
Almonds, 1 oz		3.3
Apple with skin, raw, medium		3.3
Brussel sprouts, cooked from frozen, ½ cup		3.2
Spaghetti, whole-wheat, cooked, ½ cup		3.1
Banana, medium		3.1
Orange, raw, medium		3.1
Oat bran muffin, small		3
Guava, medium		3
Pearled barley, cooked, ½ cup		3
Sauerkraut, canned, ½ cup		3
Tomato paste, ¼ cup		2.9
Winter squash, cooked, ½ cup		2.9
Broccoli, cooked, ½ cup		2.8
Parsnips, chopped, cooked, ½ cup		2.8
Turnip greens, cooked, ½ cup		2.5
Collards, cooked, ½ cup		2.7
Okra, cooked from frozen, ½ cup		2.6
Peas, edible-podded, cooked, ½ cup		2.5

Fiber Type			Fiber Containing Food
Soluble			oatmeal, oatbran
			nuts, seeds
			legumes (peas, beans and lentils)
			apple, pear, strawberry, blueberry
Insoluble			whole grains (whole wheat bread, barley, couscous, brown rice, bulgur)
			whole-grain breakfast cereal
			wheat bran
			seeds
			carrot, cucumber, zucchini, celery, tomato
Glycemic Load of Foods			Carbohydrate Containing Foods
Low (10 or under)			high fiber fruits and vegetables (but not potatoes)
			bran cereals (1 oz)
			many beans and lentils (3/4 cup or 5 oz cooked):
Medium (11 to 19)			pearled barley, cooked, 1 cup
			brown rice, cooked, ¾ cup
			oatmeal, cooked, 1 cup
			bulgur, cooked, ¾ cup
			rice cakes, 3
			whole grain bread, 1 slice
			whole grain pasta, cooked, 1¼ cup
			no-sugar added fruit juice, 8 oz
High (20 or over)			baked potato
			French fries
			cereal, refined, 1 oz
			sugar-sweetened beverage, 12 oz
			jelly beans, 10 large or 30 small
			candy bar, one 2-oz bar or 3 mini-bars
			couscous, cooked, 1 cup
			cranberry juice cocktail, 8 oz
			white basmati rice, cooked, 1 cup
			white flour pasta, cooked, 1¼ cup

Fiber Type	Fiber Containing Food
Soluble	oatmeal, oatbran
	nuts, seeds
	legumes (peas, beans and lentils)
	apple, pear, strawberry, blueberry
Insoluble	whole grains (whole wheat bread, barley, couscous, brown rice, bulgur)
	whole-grain breakfast cereal
	wheat bran
	seeds
	carrot, cucumber, zucchini, celery, tomato

Glycemic Load of Foods	Carbohydrate Containing Foods
Low (10 or under)	high fiber fruits and vegetables (but not potatoes)
	bran cereals (1 oz)
	many beans and lentils (3/4 cup or 5 oz cooked):
Medium (11 to 19)	pearled barley, cooked, 1 cup
	brown rice, cooked, ¾ cup
	oatmeal, cooked, 1 cup
	bulgur, cooked, ¾ cup
	rice cakes, 3
	whole grain bread, 1 slice
	whole grain pasta, cooked, 1¼ cup
	no-sugar added fruit juice, 8 oz
High (20 or over)	baked potato
	French fries
	cereal, refined, 1 oz
	sugar-sweetened beverage, 12 oz
	jelly beans, 10 large or 30 small
	candy bar, one 2-oz bar or 3 mini-bars
	couscous, cooked, 1 cup
	cranberry juice cocktail, 8 oz
	white basmati rice, cooked, 1 cup
	white flour pasta, cooked, 1¼ cup

Potassium Rich Foods	Potassium (mg)
Sweet potato, baked, medium	694
Tomato paste, ¼ cup	664
Beet greens, cooked, ½ cup	655
Potato, baked, 156 g	610
White beans, canned, ½ cup	595
Yogurt, plain, non-fat, 8-oz	579
Tomato puree, ½ cup	549
Clams, canned, 3 oz	534
Yogurt, plain, low-fat, 8 oz	531
Prune juice, ¾ cup	530
Carrot juice, ¾ cup	517
Halibut, cooked, 3 oz	490
Soybeans, green, cooked, ½ cup	485
Tuna, yellowfin, cooked 3 oz	484
Lima beans, cooked, ½ cup	484
Winter squash, cooked, ½ cup	448
Soybeans, mature, cooked, ½ cup	443
Rockfish, pacific, cooked, 3 oz	442
Cod, pacific, cooked, 3 oz	439
Bananas, medium	422
Spinach, cooked, ½ cup	419
Tomato juice, ¾ cup	417
Tomato sauce, ½ cup	405
Peaches, dried, uncooked, ¼ cup	398
Prunes, stewed, ½ cup	398
Milk, non-fat, 1 cup	382
Pork chop, center loin, cooked, 3 oz	382
Apricots, dried, uncooked, ¼ cup	378
Rainbow trout, farmed, cooked, 3 oz	375
Port loin, center rib roast, lean, 3 oz	371
Buttermilk, cultured, low-fat, 1 cup	370
Cantaloupe, ¼ medium	368
Milk, low-fat (1-2%), 1 cup	366
Honeydew melon, 1/8 medium	365
Lentils, cooked, ½ cup	365
Kidney beans, cooked, ½ cup	358
Orange juice, ¾ cup	355
Split peas, cooked, ½ cup	355
Yogurt, plain, whole milk, 8 oz	352

Magnesium Rich Foods (100 g uncooked)	**Magnesium Content (mg)**
Nuts and beans	**107 to 270**
Unrefined grains	**to 170**
Pumpkin seeds, roasted, 1 oz	**151**
Dark green vegetables	**25 to 105**
Chocolate (excluding milk chocolate)	120
Seafood (excluding fish)	35 to 105
Bran cereal, ready-to-eat, about 1 oz	**103**
Halibut, cooked, 3 oz	**91**
Dried fruits	55 to 90
Tuna, yellowfin, cooked, 3 oz	**54**
Artichokes (hearts), cooked, ½ cup	**50**
Tofu, firm, ½ cup	**47**
Oat bran muffin, 1 oz	45
Haddock, cooked, 3 oz	**42**

Iron Rich Foods	**Iron (mg)**
Clams, canned, drained, 3 oz	23.8
Cereal, fortified ready-to-eat, about 1 oz	1.8 to 21.1
Oysters, eastern, cooked, 3 oz	10.2
Liver (or other organ meats), cooked, 3 oz	5.2 to 9.9
Cereal, fortified instant, 1 packet	4.9 to 8.1
Soybeans, mature, cooked, ½ cup	**4.4**
Pumpkin seeds, roasted, 1 oz	**4.2**
White beans, canned, ½ cup	**3.9**
Lentils, cooked, ½ cup	**3.3**
Spinach, cooked from fresh, ½ cup	**3.2**
Beef, chuck, blade roast, lean, cooked, 3 oz	3.1
Beef, bottom round, lean, cooked, 3 oz	2.8
Kidney beans, cooked, ½ cup	**2.6**
Sardines, canned in oil, drained, 3 oz	**2.5**
Beef, rib, lean, ¼" fat, 3 oz	2.4
Chickpeas, cooked, ½ cup	**2.4**
Duck, meat only, roasted, 3 oz	2.3
Lamb, shoulder, lean with ¼" fat, cooked, 3 oz	2.3
Prune juice, ¾ cup	2.3
Shrimp, canned, 3 oz	2.3
Ground beef, 15% fat, cooked, 3 oz	2.2
Tomato puree, ½ cup	**2.2**
Lima beans, cooked, ½ cup	**2.2**
Soybeans, green, cooked, ½ cup	**2.2**
Navy beans, cooked, ½ cup	**2.1**
Refried beans, ½ cup	**2.1**
Beef, top sirloin, lean, cooked, 3 oz	2.0
Tomato paste, ¼ cup	**2.0**

Vitamin A Rich Foods	Vitamin A (retinol activity equivalents in mcg)
Liver (and other organ meats), cooked, 3 oz1490 to 9126	
Carrot juice, ¾ cup	**1692**
Sweet potato with peel, baked, medium	1096
Pumpkin, canned, ½ cup	953
Carrots, cooked from fresh, ½ cup	**671**
Spinach, cooked from frozen, ½ cup	**573**
Collards, cooked from frozen, ½ cup	**489**
Kale, cooked from frozen, ½ cup	**478**
Mixed vegetables, canned, ½ cup	**474**
Turnip greens, cooked from frozen, ½ cup	**441**
Cereal, instant cooked, fortified, 1 packet	285 to 376
Cereal, ready-to-eat, with added vitamin A, about 1 oz	180 to 376
Carrot, raw, small	**301**
Beet greens, cooked, ½ cup	**276**
Winter squash, cooked, ½ cup	**268**
Cantaloupe, raw, ¼ medium	233
Herring, pickled, 3 oz	**219**
Sweet pepper, red, cooked, ½ cup	**186**
Chinese cabbage, cooked, ½ cup	**180**

Vitamin C Rich Foods	Vitamin C (mg)
Guava, raw, ½ cup	**188**
Sweet pepper, red, raw, ½ cup	**142**
Sweet pepper, red, cooked, ½ cup	**116**
Kiwi fruit, medium	**70**
Orange, raw, medium	**70**
Orange juice, ¾ cup	61 to 93
Sweet pepper, green, raw, ½ cup	**60**
Sweet pepper, green, cooked, ½ cup	**51**
Grapefruit juice, ¾ cup	**50 to 70**
Vegetable juice cocktail, ¾ cup	50
Strawberries, raw, ½ cup	**49**
Brussel sprouts, cooked, ½ cup	**48**
Cantaloupe, ¼ medium	47
Papaya, raw, ¼ medium	47
Broccoli, raw, ½ cup	**39**
Edible pod peas, cooked, ½ cup	**38**
Broccoli, cooked, ½ cup	**37**
Sweet potato, canned, ½ cup	34
Tomato juice, ¾ cup	**33**
Cauliflower, cooked, ½ cup	**28**
Pineapple, raw, ½ cup	28
Mango, ½ cup	23

Vitamin E Rich Foods	Vitamin E (alpha-tocopherol in mg)
Cereal, fortified ready-to-eat, about 1 oz	1.6 to 12.8
Sunflower seeds, dry roasted, 1 oz	**7.4**
Almonds, 1 oz	**7.3**
Sunflower oil, 1 tbsp	**5.6**
Cottonseed oil, 1 tbsp	4.8
Safflower oil, 1 tbsp	**4.6**
Hazelnuts (filberts), 1 oz	**4.3**
Mixed nuts, dry roasted, 1 oz	**3.1**
Turnip greens, frozen, cooked, ½ cup	**2.9**
Tomato paste, ¼ cup	**2.8**
Pine nuts, 1 oz	**2.6**
Peanut butter, 2 tbsp	**2.5**
Tomato puree, ½ cup	**2.5**
Tomato sauce, ½ cup	**2.5**
Canola oil, 1 tbsp	**2.4**
Wheat germ, toasted, plain, 2 tbsp	**2.3**
Peanuts, 1 oz	**2.2**
Avocado, raw, ½	**2.1**
Carrot juice, canned, ¾ cup	**2.1**
Peanut oil, 1 tbsp	**2.1**
Corn oil, 1 tbsp	1.9
Olive oil, 1 tbsp	**1.9**
Spinach, cooked, ½ cup	**1.9**
Sardine, Atlantic, in oil, drained, 3 oz	**1.7**
Blue crab, cooked/canned, 3 oz	1.6
Brazil nuts, 1 oz	**1.6**
Herring, Atlantic, pickled, 3 oz	**1.5**

References and Suggested Readings

Center for Nutrition Policy and Promotion, US Department of Agriculture. "Dietary Guidelines for Americans 2005." www.healthierus.gov/dietaryguidelines (accessed on October 18, 2008).

Harvard School of Public Health. "The Nutrition Source." www.hsph.harvard.edu/nutritionsource (accessed February 24, 2008).

Nutrition Data. http://www.nutritiondata.com/ (accessed February 24, 2008).

Index

Made in the USA
Lexington, KY
15 September 2011